WHO Technical Report Series

Research Priorities for Zoonoses and Marginalized Infections

Technical report of the TDR Disease Reference Group on Zoonoses and Marginalized Infectious Diseases of Poverty

This report contains the collective views of an international group of experts and does not necessarily represent the decisions or the stated policy of the World Health Organization

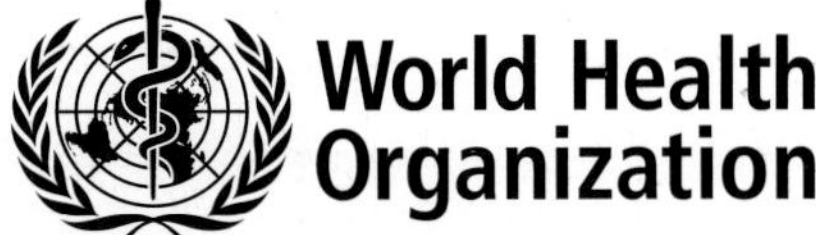

WHO Library Cataloguing-in-Publication Data

Research priorities for zoonoses and marginalized infections.

(Technical report series ; no. 971)

1. Zoonoses. 2. Research. 3. Neglected diseases. 4. Poverty. 5. Developing countries.
I.World Health Organization. II.TDR Disease Reference Group on Zoonoses and Marginalized Infectious Diseases of Poverty. III.Series.

ISBN 978 92 4 120971 7 (NLM classification: WC 950)
ISSN 0512-3054

Printed in Italy

Contents

WHO/TDR Disease Reference Group on Zoonoses and Marginalized Infectious Diseases of Poverty (DRG 6) 2009–2010

Reference Group Members

Dr H. Carabin, University of Oklahoma Health Sciences Centre, Oklahoma, OK, USA

Dr S. Cleaveland, Reader, Division of Ecology and Evolutionary Biology, University of Glasgow, Glasgow, Scotland

Dr A. Garba, Director, Réseau International Schistosomose, Environnement, Aménagement et Lutte (Riseal), Niamey, Niger

Dr E. Gotuzzo, Director, Instituto de Medicina Tropical "Alexander von Homboldt", Universidad Peruana Cayetano Heredia, Lima, Peru

Dr Z. Hallaj, Senior Consultant on communicable diseases, WHO/EMRO, Cairo, Egypt (*co-Chair*)

Dr K. Kar, Chairman, CLTS Foundation, Calcutta, India

Professor G.T. Keusch, Professor of International Health and of Medicine, Boston University, Boston, USA

Professor D.H. Molyneux, Senior Professorial Fellow, Liverpool School of Tropical Medicine, Liverpool, England (*Chair*)

Professor D.P. McManus, National Health and Medical Research Council of Australia Senior Principal Research Fellow, Head of Molecular Parasitology Laboratory, Queensland Institute of Medical Research, Brisbane, Australia

Dr H. Ngowi, Department of Veterinary Medicine and Public Health, Sokoine University of Agriculture, Morogoro, United Republic of Tanzania

Dr P. Ramos-Jimenez, Philippine NGO Council on Population Health and Welfare, Pasay City, Philippines

Dr A. Sanchez, Associate Professor, Department of Community Health Sciences, Brock University, St. Catharines, Ontario, Canada

Career Development Fellow

Dr H.M. Abushama, Assistant Professor in Immunogenetics, Department of Zoology, Faculty of Science, University of Khartoum, Khartoum, Sudan

Secretariat

Dr A. Bassili, TB Surveillance Officer and Focal Point, Tropical Disease Research, Communicable Disease Control, WHO Regional Office for the Eastern Mediterranean, Cairo, Egypt

Dr C.L. Chaignat, Medical Officer, Water, Sanitation and Hygiene, Protection of the Human Environment, WHO, Geneva, Switzerland

Dr D. Kioy, Scientist, Special Programme for Research and Training in Tropical Diseases, WHO, Geneva, Switzerland (*Manager*)

Dr F.X. Meslin, Coordinator, Neglected Zoonotic Diseases, Neglected Tropical Diseases, WHO/HQ, Geneva, Switzerland

Dr A.L. Willingham, Scientist, Special Programme for Research and Training in Tropical Diseases, WHO, Geneva, Switzerland

Abbreviations

AE	alveolar echinococcosis
BNP	Blue Nile Health Project
CE	cystic echinococcosis
CLTS	Community-led Total Sanitation
CNS	Central Nervous System
CT	Computerized axial Tomography
DALY	disability-adjusted life year
DRG	Disease Reference Group
EMRO	WHO Regional Office for the Eastern Mediterranean
EPEC	enteropathogenic *E.coli*
ETEC	enterotoxigenic *E.coli*
FAO	Food and Agriculture Organization of the United Nations
FBT	foodborne trematodiasis
GAVI	Global Alliance for Vaccines and Immunization
GBD	global burden of disease
GFATM	Global Fund to Fight AIDS, Tuberculosis and Malaria
GMP	Good Manufacturing Practice
HAART	highly active antiretroviral therapy
HALY	health-adjusted life years
IMCI	Integrated Management of Childhood Illness
MDA	mass drug administration
MDGs	Millennium Development Goals
MRI	Magnetic Resonance Imaging
NCC	neurocysticercosis
NTD	neglected tropical disease
NZD	neglected zoonotic disease
ODA	Official Development Assistance
ODF	open defecation free

OIE	Office International des Epizooties (World Organization for Animal Health)
OVD	oral vaccination of dogs
PCR	Polymerase chain reaction
PEP	post-exposure prophylaxis
QALY	quality-adjusted life years
TDPS	Target-driven Partial Sanitation
TRG	Thematic Reference Group
USDA	Unites States Department of Agriculture

Details on The Global Report for Research on Infectious Disease of Poverty can be found at http://www.who.int/tdr/stewardship/global_report/en/index.html

Executive Summary

The Disease Reference Group on Zoonoses and Marginalized Infectious Diseases of Poverty (DRG6) was part of an independent think tank of international experts, established by the Special Programme for Research and Training in Tropical Diseases (TDR) to identify key research priorities through the review of research evidence and input from stakeholder consultations.

Context

There has been limited recognition by the global health community that zoonoses and marginalized infectious diseases are major causes of poverty and thus constraints on development. A Disease Reference Group (DRG) was created to review the zoonotic diseases and these marginalized infectious diseases and to provide an analysis of research priorities. The report emphasizes that the diseases discussed are diverse and cover the spectrum of infectious agents, from viruses to worms. The infections display a variety of transmission patterns, have a global geographical distribution throughout the tropics and subtropics, and exist in different ecological environments and in different health system settings. However, this complexity is compounded, compared with non-zoonotic infections, by the need to involve other sectors (for example livestock services, education, environment, water and sanitation, and wildlife) when decisions on policy for control, financing for control across sectors, defining research priorities and implementing research findings are made.

The Group also highlighted cross-disease and thematic issues following interaction between members, stakeholders and the WHO Secretariat. A series of matrices was developed to evaluate the priorities from the perspective of cross-cutting themes for research. This approach was designed to recognize the complexity of the priority-setting task and to highlight the challenges of implementation of research findings where zoonotic diseases are not accorded high priority as they primarily affect marginalized populations with limited access to government services. The Group also recognized that two levels of prioritization were necessary. Firstly, disease-specific and focused priorities were addressed, driven by the appropriate biomedical or social paradigm. These recommendations are extensive and relevant to disease-focused scientific constituencies. Secondly, broader priorities emerged that are relevant to the different diseases considered in this report and infectious diseases in general.

Disease-specific priorities

Biomedical priorities were identified for specific diseases and drew on the expert opinions of the DRG and stakeholder discussions, as well as existing published material from WHO and other authoritative groups, including disease-specific partnerships. These priorities were grouped into the needs for new drugs, diagnostics, and human and animal vaccines.

Macro priorities for policy-makers

Common priorities emerged irrespective of the disease entity or infectious agent being addressed. Stakeholders highlighted significant issues that require emphasis. For example, in many countries a large proportion of the population is dependent on livestock for its social and economic well-being, and in these countries a high proportion of the Gross Domestic Product is derived from livestock production. Therefore, the report identified what it termed macro priorities, covering all the diseases included in the analysis. These are:

- expand the surveillance for zoonotic diseases in humans and animals;
- re-attribute the burden of morbidity and mortality attributed to diseases and conditions (cancers, neurological conditions, injuries) to the neglected parasitic/zoonotic diseases;
- re-evaluate the societal burden of disease for zoonoses;
- expand systems research to determine how best the different sectors can interact;
- evaluate the effectiveness of community-led approaches, including the Community-led Total Sanitation approach, in the control of zoonotic infectious diseases;
- integrate animal and human disease expertise with social science perspectives;
- conduct more extensive studies on the costs of intervention, the cost–benefits and cost–effectiveness;
- scale up research training to increase human resources in the area of public health, including veterinary and livestock services, for addressing zoonoses;
- create opportunities to evaluate and modify control strategies as experience is gained in implementation;
- combine interventions allied to improved water and sanitation, and health education and promotion, and deploy them for the human and animal diseases in parallel;
- expand research on the use of new communication technologies such as smart phones to enhance surveillance, reporting and evaluation.

The conclusions and deliberations of the DRG are summarized in Figure 1. They specify the disease-specific priorities versus the broader macro priorities.

Figure 1
Research priorities for zoonotic diseases

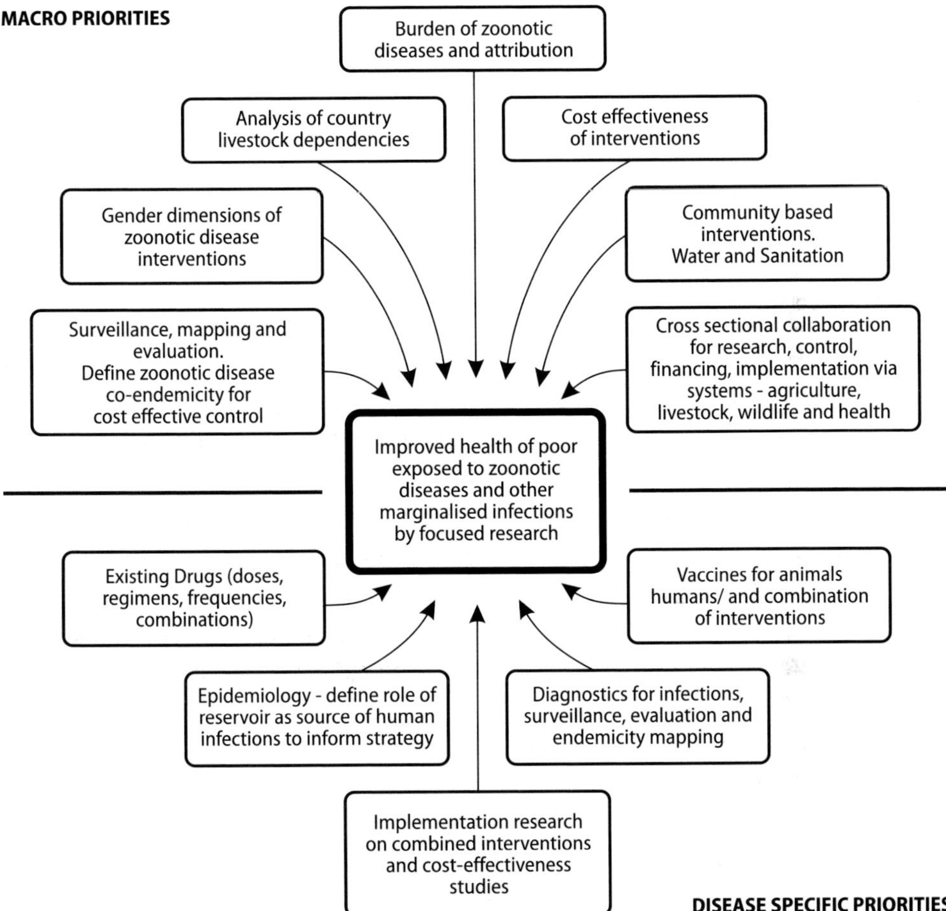

1. Introduction

As part of its ten-year strategy[1] to foster "an effective global research effort on infectious diseases of poverty in which disease-endemic countries play a pivotal role", TDR established a global research think tank of 125 international experts to continually and systematically review evidence, assess research needs and, following periodic national and regional stakeholder consultations, set research priorities for accelerating the control of infectious diseases of poverty. Working in ten disease-specific and thematic reference groups (DRGs/TRGs), these experts were crucial contributors to TDR's stewardship mandate for the acquisition and analysis of information on infectious diseases of poverty[2]. Their work is ultimately intended to promote control-relevant research, achieve research innovation and enhance the capacity of disease-endemic countries to resolve public health problems related to the disproportionate burden of infectious diseases among the poor.

This report addresses the research needs of zoonotic diseases (the diseases of animals that also affect humans) as well as other marginalized infections of some of the world's poorest people and communities, often living beyond the reach of the formal health system. Research priorities identified by the Reference Group on Zoonoses and Marginalized Infectious Diseases (DRG6) are presented in this report.

1.1 Rationale and context

The majority of infectious diseases mainly affect poor and marginalized populations that lack access to health services and are readily ignored. As a result, these populations are subjected to a cycle of ill-health and poverty that aggravates their burden of infectious diseases. Of some 1400 species of infectious disease pathogens of humans, nearly 60% are derived from animal sources, hence the importance of recognizing the role of livestock, companion animals and wildlife in the interactions between animals and humans (*1*, *2*). In addition two thirds of emerging pathogens are of zoonotic origin (*1*, *2*). Only by recognizing the importance of these human–animal interactions can we fully understand how to control these infections.

Zoonotic diseases, although biologically diverse, share common characteristics associated with the conditions under which poor people live in the world's poorest countries. These features are usually the result of social, economic, geographical and political forces. We have an excellent understanding

[1] Details on TDR's strategy can be found at http://www.who.int/tdr/about/strategy/strategy_06.htm

[2] Details on TDR's stewardship function can be found at http://www.who.int/tdr/about/strategy/business_plan.pdf, pp. 18-21

of the biological features of the etiology, transmission and epidemiology of a particular infection, but reducing the burden of disease must be undertaken in communities and populations within the framework of local or national settings and through coordinated policy.

Recent pandemic threats have raised concern in developed countries, as their populations and economies are threatened. In response, developed countries have provided significant resources for targeted surveillance and control of these emerging global problems. Most of these intermittent global threats have emerged from animal sources. However, many marginalized populations are living in close contact with animals on a daily basis since they are dependent on livestock as a critical resource for survival. They are thus exposed, together with their livestock, to debilitating infections through the frequency of their contacts. History has shown that infections constantly emerge from animal populations. Such threats have always provoked fear, fueled in recent years by the emergence of HIV, Ebola, Nipah, Lassa, SARS, H5N1 and H1N1 influenza viruses, and *E. coli* O157:H7, all of animal origin.

The number of people who are directly dependent on livestock is estimated at some 600 million, nearly a tenth of the world's population, and in more marginal lands of the tropics the proportion of the population so dependent can be as high as 70%. However, for effective disease control, the zoonotic diseases need multisectoral collaboration between the human and veterinary health, agricultural, and water and sanitation sectors.

A further feature of zoonotic and marginalized diseases is that they predominate among populations living in conflict and war zones, internally displaced populations, refugees, and those affected by natural disasters (earthquakes, volcanoes and tsunamis). In such situations, already weak infrastructures for health and limited resources cannot cope with the increased burden of infectious diseases, even though the pattern of emergence of diseases in these situations is well known.

In environments where zoonotic diseases represent a high burden, health systems are weak, fragmented or not accessible to populations living "beyond the end of the road". Hence there is inadequate surveillance and reporting of disease outbreaks, a situation compounded by inadequate diagnostic and therapeutic services. In addition, the efficacy of drugs for both humans and animals is not effectively monitored as a result of lack of control of imports and the widespread sale of ineffective or counterfeit products through an unregulated private sector.

A sizeable proportion of the burden of zoonotic disease seems likely to result from endemic, chronic, disabling, frequently misdiagnosed and often unreported infections of remote populations that are dependent on livestock for their survival and asset base. Such populations, often nomadic, have limited contact with or access to formal health services and live beyond the reach of surveillance systems. This report seeks to bridge this human–animal interface by linking research knowledge to the control of zoonoses of human public health and veterinary public health importance. It seeks to provide stakeholders with a greater understanding of the opportunities of a strategic vision of the research needed to diminish the impact of these infections. The report emphasizes that, in many low-income countries, a high proportion of the total population is dependent on livestock and that a significant proportion of the Gross Domestic Product is derived from livestock. In the humid savannas and forests of sub-Saharan Africa, the consumption of game meat or "bushmeat" represents a major source of protein, with the attendant risks of the acquisition of a variety of pathogens due to the exposure of humans to animal species ranging from rodents and bats to non-human primates.

Infectious diseases affect the poorest people on the planet, those who have been called "the bottom billion" (*3*, *4*). Addressing one disease at a time means that attention to their control has depended on donor priority ratings on the one hand and on the power of advocacy constituencies on the other. As a result the Global Fund to Fight AIDS, Tuberculosis, and Malaria (GFATM) was established as a financing mechanism to coordinate donor efforts and to ensure efficient distribution of financial resources. One consequence has been greater overall resources for these three diseases, at the potential expense of stagnant investments in other highly prevalent diseases of poverty with arguably a higher overall burden than the specific diseases addressed by GFATM (*4*).

1.2 Zoonoses and the Millennium Development Goals

Zoonoses are not overtly mentioned in the Millennium Development Goals (MDGs) and therefore are relegated to the basket of "other diseases" included in MDG 6, which is primarily focused on HIV and malaria. However, as this report shows, the zoonotic diseases have a profound impact on the health of the poorest, whose sole source of income and only asset is often their livestock. A stakeholder meeting in Cairo, Egypt, highlighted the arid zones of sub-Saharan Africa and the Eastern Mediterranean Region, where the loss of the traditional systems of livestock husbandry through drought, animal or human disease, ecological stress or civil unrest has threatened the very existence of these communities, which are critically dependent on the well-being of their livestock. These communities are often marginalized not only through the stresses described above but also by political, social, cultural and economic forces. They are often minority ethnic groups, are migratory and traditionally do not participate in mainstream education, and they lack access to any government service. Although the zoonotic diseases themselves are not specified within the framework of the MDGs, addressing diseases of poverty, both in humans and animals, will have an impact on the success of ongoing and future attempts to improve the lives of the poorest populations in the poorest countries. Ensuring the health of the livestock has further implications for the maintenance of the rural economy, as many infections of livestock have an impact on their productivity in terms of milk or meat output, animal value at slaughter, loss of manure as a fertilizer, and reduced income from sale of livestock. In addition, in many societies, smallholder farming is under the control of women, who can suffer disproportionately from the adverse consequences of human and/or animal disease, through loss of income and hence loss of independence. The benefits in the context of MDGs relating to maternal and child health and access to health and education can thus be traced to the effective maintenance of the traditional way of life, assured through the health of livestock in these populations, particularly in arid environments.

The "other diseases" of MDG 6 which include the even more neglected zoonoses, need to be re-addressed in the context of what may be gained in terms of poverty alleviation through implementation of cost-effective interventions on the one hand and more focused research on the other. The "other diseases" (except tuberculosis, which was included in GFATM) and perhaps polio eradication have remained secondary priorities, despite accumulating evidence for the effectiveness of control measures that can be deployed at the population level and the knowledge that over one billion people are infected and some 2.7 billion are probably at risk of "other diseases" besides the "big three" (*3–5*). For the zoonotic diseases, there is a need for stronger advocacy and for a focused research agenda directed at improved approaches to control. As suggested by Molyneux (*4*), while the 10/90 gap in research efforts (referring to the fact that less than 10% of global funding is devoted to 90% of the world's health problems) is well defined, this gap for the most neglected diseases is probably closer to 1/99. Such a ratio certainly applies to the zoonotic diseases where the burden:research ratio was not calculated by a study of the research spending on neglected diseases (*6*).

The comparative lack of research investment in diseases other than the "big three" diseases of poverty, and the disparity between burden of disease and investment has been well documented (*6*). It has been calculated that the total investment in neglected tropical disease control (excluding HIV/TB and malaria) is only 0.6% of total Official Development Assistance (ODA) funding for health, despite the large population of infected and very poor people at risk (*7*).

1.3 Challenges

The most important initial observation is that there is limited reliable qualitative and quantitative information on the burden of zoonotic diseases, as well as a lack of information on their geographical (regional) distribution in endemic countries. One of the challenges in estimating burden of disease is the weak health and agricultural information systems in endemic countries, including the lack of reporting (or underreporting) of infectious diseases. Similarly, because of limited national government expenditures for health, surveillance remains particularly underfunded, which limits the ability to estimate reliably the burden of these infections. Limited funding also handicaps control of zoonotic diseases as the interaction between those responsible for human health, animal health and wildlife services is impeded, leading to the failure to identify disease outbreaks and contributing to the limited awareness of zoonotic infections at the policy level. Because zoonotic diseases often occur in communities beyond the reach of the formal health facilities, education systems and livestock services, reporting and certification of deaths may not be possible. This information is a prerequisite for the acquisition of accurate data upon which the Global Burden of Disease Studies depend.

Inadequate surveillance and reporting are characteristic of zoonoses, and many zoonotic infections have clinical manifestations, being characterized only by febrile episodes. Some diseases, however, can be stigmatizing and are hence kept hidden. For example, neurocysticercosis is associated with a range of symptoms, such as epileptic seizures and severe chronic headaches, while liver fluke infections with opisthorchiasis and clonorchiasis can lead to bile duct carcinomas. Moreover, the definitive diagnosis for several of these helminth infections requires advanced techniques such as imaging, which are rarely available and are unaffordable in the settings where the zoonoses are a major burden. Clusters of cases and their true etiology may also go unrecognized, especially if they occur in isolated areas. This leads to a further underestimation of their incidence, the starting point for assessing disease burden. The lack of information on the social and economic outcomes of zoonoses, including the direct (treatment costs) and indirect (productivity losses) costs in both humans and animals, and the indirect impact of reduced productivity in livestock (meat, milk, manure), remain a serious deficit. The fact that zoonoses can affect in turn the cash value of animals and reduce the availability of protein, contributing to malnutrition, growth reduction and cognitive deficits, remains a serious and systemic deficit.

At the national level, countries where zoonoses are endemic have limited qualified human resources to deal with the challenges of control of infectious diseases. In ministries of health, the personnel dealing with surveillance and research may have limited experience with zoonoses. In addition, epidemiologists and health economists who work in local academic institutions, have other responsibilities that limit the time they can devote to collaboration with governmental agencies.

At the international level, considerable resources are now devoted to combating HIV, malaria, tuberculosis, poliomyelitis and vaccine-preventable diseases through GFATM, the Global Polio Eradication Initiative and the Global Alliance for Vaccines and Immunization (GAVI). In contrast, until recently, there has been little attention to the neglected tropical diseases (NTDs) that are most prevalent among the bottom billion on the socioeconomic ladder (*3*). In addition, in most of the disease-endemic countries, research agendas do not prioritize the challenges faced by the disease control programmes, in large part because they are usually set by academic institutions without addressing or seeking to influence the national priorities in disease control.

1.4 Scope of the report

The comparative lack of research investment in neglected diseases other than the "big three" diseases of poverty, and the disparity between burden of disease and investment have been documented (*6*). It has been calculated that the total investment in neglected tropical disease control (excluding HIV/TB and malaria) is only 0.6% of total Official Development Assistance (ODA) funding for health, despite the over one billion people considered to be at risk (*7*). This report examines zoonotic and marginalized diseases caused by an array of diverse infective agents, from viruses to worms, with very different transmission mechanisms, epidemiology, geographical distribution, control interventions, evaluation and surveillance procedures. This diversity of agents creates a further dimension – the need to bring together new constituencies of stakeholders working across the animal-human interface and provides a unique challenge in priority setting.

This report focuses on the following specific infections:

1) **Helminth infections**
   - taeniasis/cysticercosis
   - echinococcosis
   - zoonotic schistosomiasis
   - foodborne trematodiases

2) **Protozoan infections**
   - toxoplasmosis
   - cryptosporidiosis

3) **Bacterial infections**
   - brucellosis
   - enteric infections
   - bovine tuberculosis
   - anthrax

4) **Viral infections**
   - rabies

This report did not consider rotavirus infection because, while it is a cause of high morbidity and mortality, it is already receiving considerable attention elsewhere. Effective vaccines are now available and will probably be deployed widely in the coming years. The remaining diarrhoeal diseases are particularly linked to poverty with its attendant limited access to safe water and sanitation facilities, and inadequate access to health services. These infections are considered in this report, particularly as they relate to and enhance the cost–effectiveness of ecosystem, water supply and sanitation improvements that can reduce the burden of diarrhoeal and other infectious agents, whether zoonotic in nature or not.

1.5 Group membership

The Disease Reference Group on Zoonoses and Marginalized Infectious Diseases of Poverty (DRG 6) consisted of 13 experts in the area of zoonotic diseases and cross-cutting themes (Appendix 1). Members were identified from research institutions, international organizations, bilateral institutions, health and medical organizations, and governmental and inter-governmental organizations worldwide. Particular attention was paid to the geographical distribution, to ensure disease-endemic country and regional input as well as technical input, and gender balance of the membership. Members were formally appointed by the Director, TDR, for an initial period of two years. All members were obliged to declare any conflict of interest and confidentiality.

The Chair and co-Chair of the group were selected on the basis of their internationally-recognized research and control experience in disease-endemic countries.

1.6 Host country

To ensure that the countries most affected by diseases of poverty contribute to, and share ownership of the research agenda emerging from this initiative, the Reference Groups were hosted by disease-endemic countries, in partnership with WHO country and regional offices (Appendix 2).

The DRG was hosted in the WHO Regional Office for the Eastern Mediterranean (EMRO), Cairo Egypt.

1.7 Think tank members

The think tank was designed to draw on the best expertise internationally (Appendix 3), and to maximize partnerships with countries most affected by diseases of poverty. The 10 Reference Groups making up the think tank included researchers and public health experts from the most affected countries, and these countries also hosted the Groups. WHO country and regional offices supported both the Reference Groups and broad-based stakeholder consultations (Appendix 4).

2. Methodology and prioritization

A preliminary informal consultation was convened by TDR in Geneva to discuss the broad issues of the diseases that the DRG, when formally established, would address. This meeting was necessary as TDR had not previously been involved in these diseases, yet zoonotic diseases represented significant challenges in terms of their impact and burden on the poor in endemic countries. The DRG on Zoonoses and Marginalized Infectious Diseases (DRG 6) was thus established to prepare a status report on research into these infections and provide input for the Global Report for Research on Infectious Diseases of Poverty[1].

The purpose of DRG 6 was to systematically review research evidence and evaluate its relevance to control needs, assess challenges in control and highlight new and significant scientific advances. It was also to provide independent advice and guidance on priority areas and critical research gaps as a contribution to the Global Report. It is recognized that there are many ways to identify priorities based on expected outcomes. DRG 6 followed a sequential strategy, starting with initial informal consultation, semiquantitative prioritization exercises by members followed by a further stakeholders' consultation, proceeding to the development of a series of matrices based on specific indicators of identified research priorities. The DRG also drew on authoritative reports, some of which were convened under the auspices of WHO and TDR, which had also identified priorities for some of the diseases discussed.

2.1 Informal consultation

An informal consultation to discuss the scope, framework and membership of a DRG on infectious diseases associated with poverty including zoonoses other than those in the "traditional" TDR disease portfolio was held 2–3 June 2009 in Geneva. The consultation had the following specific objectives: 1) to define and agree on criteria for selecting the infectious diseases and research areas of the DRG; 2) to determine the scope of the DRG (diseases and research areas), and 3) to recommend potential membership of the DRG based on the scope of the mandate, skill sets and expertise required. Members of the informal consultation included experts on a variety of relevant diseases and specialities from WHO and countries (representative of all WHO regions). The Group then discussed and defined the disease scope and categories for the thematic analytical work.

2.2 Selection of DRG members

Potential members were identified from research institutions, international organizations, health and medical organizations, and governmental and inter-

[1] http://www.who.int/tdr/stewardship/global_report/en/index.html

governmental organizations worldwide. An initial list of 45 experts selected on the basis of the following required matching expertise: veterinary public health, veterinary laboratory science, wildlife biology, health social sciences (medical anthropologist/community health), clinical medicine (infectious diseases experts), water and sanitation, parasitology/microbiology/genomics and genetics, health/agriculture economics and diagnostics, was prepared and subjected to voting by a panel of WHO internal and external researchers. Particular attention was paid to the geographical distribution, to ensure disease-endemic country and regional input as well as technical input, and gender balance of the membership. The final list of 13 members was formally appointed by the Director, TDR for an initial period of two years. All members were obliged to declare any conflict of interest and confidentiality.

2.3 First DRG meeting

Following the selection of DRG members and in preparation for the first meeting in November 2009, members were asked to prepare and present the research issues in their areas of expertise. All the identified areas were discussed in detail and a list of diseases on which to focus was identified. Following the first meeting of the DRG, members initiated report writing within their areas of expertise, and a draft report was created to be discussed at a stakeholders' consultation.

2.4 Stakeholders' consultations

Periodic regional and national stakeholders' consultations are an essential part of the analytical process, enabling validation, endorsement and uptake of final research priorities, and ensuring that the work of the DRG is authoritative, scientifically credible and relevant for policy.

The stakeholders' consultation was organized by WHO/EMRO, the DRG host, to discuss the scope, relevance, research gaps and validation of research priorities. It was held in Cairo, Egypt, on 29 March 2010. Regional and national stakeholder consultations based in endemic countries represented an essential part of the analytical process.

Key stakeholders included the ministers of health, other representatives of the ministries of health, ministers of agriculture and animal resources of Egypt, Sudan and Yemen, who emphasized the importance of research in these diseases where there is an interface between humans and animals. They endorsed the concept note and provided input in the identification of research priorities in relation to real needs in their countries. Other participants included international organization (OIE), academic institutions (Imperial College London, University of KwaZulu-Natal, University of Costa Rica, the National Autonomous University of Honduras) and representatives of WHO regions.

2.5 Second DRG meeting

As a result of the stakeholders' consultation discussions, a semiquantitative matrix system was developed during the second DRG meeting in order to ensure that cross-cutting issues relevant to each specific disease were considered and to indicate a priority rating. The meeting took place in Cairo, Egypt, the DRG's host country, from 30 to 31 March 2010.

2.6 Prioritization process

The disease-specific priorities were derived from expert opinion of the DRG, as formulated by previous relevant WHO/HQ and regional meetings and WHO/TDR meetings on the different disease groups, from peer-reviewed papers from experts and from prominent publications that had policy relevance. The DRG was also cognizant of funding bodies that had an interest in the diseases considered by the group, including disease-specific regional working groups, the OIE and the research focus of these organizations.

During its meetings and via electronic communication, the DRG identified research priorities for both individual diseases and the broader intervention-based approaches, which require cross-cutting social science research particularly in areas of health education and promotion, community-based approaches and operational research required to scale up existing strategies for zoonotic disease control. The stakeholders' consultation was also presented with the initial broad conclusions of the DRG and endorsed the approach the DRG had taken and the initial view of the priorities identified. The DRG also highlighted a multiplicity of cross-disease and thematic issues that emerged during intensive debate and interaction between members, stakeholders and the Secretariat.

Following its initial scan of priorities during and after its first meeting, the DRG developed a structured approach and methodology for addressing priorities based on the experience of the members and the feedback from wider discussions. The report is based on this accumulated experience and knowledge of the health, livestock and education sectors from both a research and an implementation perspective. The priorities were examined in a semiquantitative way. This allowed a multidimensional approach where the diseases, the cross-cutting topics and the interventions could be addressed and prioritized. This enabled scores to be analysed and rated on a scale of 1-5 (5 being the highest priority level). The analysis led to the identification of priorities shown in Figure 1 as macro and disease-specific priorities. At the end of the process, the DRG published a summary of priorities identified for zoonoses and marginalized infectious diseases of poverty (*8*).

2.7 Transformation of DRG report to TRS

The process of finalization of the report and its transformation into a publication in the WHO Technical Report Series was carried out through electronic communication between the Chair, co-Chair, DRG members and the Secretariat. The Secretariat undertook the organization of external and internal reviews of the report, and comments on structure and content were addressed in the final version of the report.

This report was assessed by the WHO Guidelines Review Committee, which recommended that it be published as an Expert Report.

3. Burden of disease

Disease burden is defined as the "size of a health problem in an area, measured by cost, mortality, morbidity or other indicators". This definition clearly shows that disease burden may be captured by different measures, which are described in the following section.

3.1 Estimating the burden of parasitic zoonoses: approaches and challenges

The various methods that may be used to estimate disease burden in animals and humans are summarized in Table 1 (9).

Table 1
Comparisons of the main measures of disease burden

Measure of burden	Items	Availability / quality of data	
		Humans	Animals
Mortality	Cause-specific death rates	Quality highly variable between countries	Rarely available except for notifiable diseases.
Morbidity	Disease-specific incidence rates	Notifiable / registry disease data Quality / completeness highly variable.	Research studies only Acute, non-recurrent and notifiable diseases (i.e. rabies) if denominator known
	Disease-specific prevalence	National / special survey data Special survey data often provide overestimate	Slaughterhouse data where home slaughtering is rare Special survey data often provide overestimate
QALYs	Cause-specific death rates	Quality highly variable between countries	Not applicable
	Life expectancy	Largely available	
	Disease-specific incidence rates	Notifiable / registry disease data. Quality / completeness highly variable.	

continues

Table 1 *continued*

Measure of burden	Items	Availability / quality of data	
		Humans	**Animals**
QALYs	Time evolution of disease states	Knowledge of natural history of disease needed	Not applicable
	Quality of life measure at various disease states	Special studies. Place/time specific	
DALYs	Cause-specific death rates	Quality highly variable between countries	Not applicable
	Disease-specific incidence rates	Notifiable / registry disease data. Quality / completeness highly variable.	
	Distribution of sequelae associated with disease in treatment-free individuals	Knowledge of natural history of disease needed	
	Duration of each sequela in treatment-free individuals	Knowledge of natural history of each sequela needed	
	Distribution of sequelea associated with disease among people under treatment	Special studies required	
	Duration of each sequela under treatment	Special studies required	
	Disability weights for each sequela (treated / non-treated)	Available from GBD initiative. Not all sequelae have been attributed disability weights	

continues

Table 1 *continued*

Measure of burden	Items	Availability / quality of data	
		Humans	Animals
Monetary burden	Cause-specific death rates	Quality highly variable between countries	Rarely available except for notifiable diseases.
	Disease-specific prevalence	National / special survey data Special survey data often provide overestimate	Slaughterhouse data where home slaughtering is rare Special survey data often provide overestimate
	Distribution of sequelae associated with disease	Knowledge of natural history of disease needed	Knowledge of natural history of disease needed
	Frequency of care / treatments / diagnoses and productivity losses for each sequela	Special studies Expert opinion	Special studies Expert opinion
	Costs associated with care / treatments / productivity losses of each sequela	Country-level health / labour statistics Special surveys	Agricultural statistics Special surveys

3.1.1 Measures of mortality, morbidity and health-associated life years

3.1.1.1 Measures of mortality and morbidity in humans

Several methods have been proposed to compare the burden of human diseases worldwide. The traditional method has been to use cause-specific death rates (*10*). The reported advantage of this approach is the availability of death certificates worldwide. However, the determination of the cause of death as listed on death certificates has been shown to be poor in a number of countries (*11*).

Many demographers would dispute the claim that death certification is available widely. In remote communities where zoonoses are prevalent, the existence of a death certification process and/or an accurate assessment of the cause of death is unlikely. This is particularly the case where death is followed traditionally by burial within 24 hours. Moreover, in cases of death reporting, other errors can arise, such as;

1) ignorance of all diseases that are not fatal but may contribute to a fatal outcome due to another cause;
2) underestimation of the prevalence of common diseases that are rarely fatal;
3) underestimation of the distal rather than proximal causes of death, such as underlying nutritional status, reduced immunological status or co-morbidity.

Another option is to measure the frequency of occurrence of each disease. Such data can originate from surveillance systems, public health records or specific studies where medical charts are reviewed. The most commonly available data are those from surveillance systems. Surveillance systems, however, have several limitations. These include:

1) variation in the quality and completeness of the data from country to country and within a country from region to region;
2) the limited number of diseases under surveillance and covered by the reporting systems;
3) inclusion of only those cases that are reported to the authorities.

This leads to a poor representation of the true frequency of specific diseases and prevents the development of accurate maps of disease prevalence.

3.1.1.2 Measures of health-associated life years in humans

Measuring the prevalence of a particular disease does not capture associated duration, suffering and subsequent disability. Such impacts of disease can be measured with health-adjusted life years (HALYs). The two most common HALYs are quality-adjusted life years (QALYs) and disability-adjusted life years (DALYs). Several multi-attribute measurement tools have been developed to link a health measurement scale to utility of health values. The most commonly used measurement scales are the Quality of Health Being (QHB), the Health Utilities Index (HUI), the Short Form series (SF) and the Euro-Qol series *(12)*. These scales measure several aspects of functioning (i.e. physical, social, mental). Questionnaires are used to calculate a score, which is correlated with utility values, used to compare the impact of diseases.

Food safety issues and restrictions to trade

Outbreaks of zoonotic diseases can lead to disruption in local markets and may result in the restriction of movement of animals (2). Barriers to export markets have less impact on most rural communities. However where goods are exported there is a multiplier effect on employment and auxiliary sectors leading to a much amplified effect on whole communities (2).

Conservation issues

Neglected zoonotic disease (NZD) may cause mortality in wild animals leading to extinction of endangered species (e.g. African wild dogs from rabies). This could also have an impact on the ability to generate income in communities that rely on tourism.

3.1.3 Case-studies

3.1.3.1 The monetary burden of cysticercosis

There are significant agricultural losses related to *Taenia solium* infection of pigs caused by cystic stages of the parasite. Porcine cysticercosis often results in total condemnation of pig carcasses since pigs can harbour thousands of cysts, making the meat from these animals unsafe to eat. Pig traders, aware of the disease, may detect infection during a pre-purchase examination and then refuse to buy a suspect pig. Farms and whole communities may become stigmatized when they are known to sell infected pigs and/or cyst-contaminated meat. Several studies have assessed the monetary burden due to cysticercosis infection, as shown in Table 2 (*19–22*). A pig carcass infected with cysticercosis is sold at a decreased price, which can vary from 25% of the usual market price in Benin to 50% in Rwanda (*20*). There is also a loss of profit when farmers do not sell their meat to official markets (*17*).

The combined cost of cysticercosis in humans and animals has been estimated in two countries (*17, 23*). The proportion of epilepsy cases attributable to neurocysticercosis (NCC) and the proportion of working time lost were found to have the most influence on the estimated monetary burden (*23*).

3.1.3.2 The monetary burden of cystic echinococcosis

The combined human and animal monetary burden of cystic echinococcosis has been estimated from several countries. One limitation mentioned in all the studies has been the lack of knowledge of the impact of infection in people without obvious symptoms and the estimates of the reduction in productivity in animals. The monetary impact of cystic echinococcosis has been evaluated in a number of countries; the results are reported in Table 3. Although these studies vary in the methods used, they provide a broad estimate of the costs of cystic echinococcosis.

Table 2
Summary of monetary burden of cystcercosis

Monetary Loss	Country	Cause	Equivalent	Reference
≥ US$ 120 million annually	China	cysticercosis infection	Amount of pork discarded 200 million kg	(*22*)
US$ 9.0–32.3 to US$ 12.8–70.0 million depending on the methods used	Eastern Cape Province, South Africa	NCC-associated epilepsy, benefits from pork not sold in slaughterhouses (2004)	5–10% of the annual health expenditures (US$ 41.3 per capita)	(*17*)
€6.9–14.8 million	West Cameroon	NCC-associated epilepsy and 30% loss of value for infected pig carcases (year unknown)	5.6% of per capita expenditure on health (2004) (US$ 44)	(*23*)
US$ 996 per case for the first 2 years of treatment	Lima, Peru	49 NCC patients residing in Lima treated in a neurological reference hospital (1999-2002)	54% of minimal wage during the first year of treatment; 16% of minimal wage during the second year of treatment	(*24*)
US$ 174.7 per patient	Andhra Pradesh, India	Solitary Cyst Granuloma NCC-associated new onset seizures patients in a seizure clinic (1997)	50.9% of per capita GDP	(*25*)
US$ 2.1–14.0 million per year; average $56 500 per hospitalization)	Los Angeles, CA, USA	3,618 hospitalized NCC adult cases (1991–2002)	Average per NCC hospitalization almost twice average US hospitalization (US$ 24 000)	(*26*)

Table 3
Summary of monetary burden of cystic echinococcosis

Country (year of valuation)	Estimated annual societal monetary burden	% agricultural monetary burden	References
Jordan (unknown)	US$ 3.9 million	92%	(*27*)
Wales, United Kingdom (1997)	US$ 1.1–6.7 million	73–76%	(*28*)
Uruguay (unknown)	US$ 2.9–22.1 million	16–70%	(*29*)
Tunisia (2000)	US$ 10.7–14.7 million	56–57%	(*18*)
China (unknown)	US$ 0.94 million	97%	(*30*)
Spain (2005)	US$ 19.5–184.6 million	10–95%	(*31*)
Global burden	US$ 4.1 billion	46% human treatment, 54% animal health costs	http://www.who.int/neglected_diseases/2010report/en/index.html

3.1.3.3 The monetary burden of rabies

The monetary burden of rabies has been estimated for Africa and Asia, including data on the costs of post-exposure prophylaxis (PEP), costs relating to the control of dog rabies (dog vaccination and population control), rabies surveillance costs and livestock losses (*15*). In this analysis, the direct medical costs include the cost of biological reagents (rabies vaccines and immunoglobulin) and their administration (including materials and staff salaries). Indirect costs represent 50% of total costs (*32*) and include transport costs to and from treatment centres and loss of income while receiving treatment in the case of both bite victims and their accompanying adults.

The monetary burden of rabies in Africa and Asia was estimated as US$ 583 (90% CI: 540–626) million (*33*), but this is considered an underestimate for several reasons. Firstly, it is recognized that the number of vaccine doses used has been widely underestimated owing to a lack of data from many countries. Secondly, vaccine and travel costs have been estimated conservatively (US$ 40 per PEP course in Africa and US$ 49 in Asia). Moreover, shortages of PEP, which occur frequently, increase costs as bite victims are required to travel elsewhere for treatment (*34*).

Thirdly, livestock losses have been estimated on the basis of laboratory sample submissions, which are also likely to be a gross underestimate, even with correction for assumed underreporting. In a detailed contact-tracing study in northern United Republic of Tanzania, livestock deaths were 2–5 times higher than figures used in an analysis, with an incidence of 12–25 deaths/100 000 cattle/year (*15, 32*). Finally, this analysis did not include income loss resulting from premature deaths, which dominates any evaluation of economic burden due to the high childhood mortality associated with rabies. According to these estimates, the economic burden of rabies for Africa and Asia is more than US$ 3 billion. The monetary burden of rabies is summarized in Table 4.

Table 4
Summary of monetary burden of rabies

Monetary loss In US$	Country	Cause	Reference
563 (520–605.8) million	Asia	Post–exposure treatment and dog rabies control costs	(*15, 32*)
20.5 (19.3–21.8) million	Africa	Post–exposure treatment and dog rabies control costs	(*15 ,32*)
300 million	USA	Prevention	(*33*)
> 4 billion	Global	Prevention and control, plus income loss due to premature deaths	http://www.rabiescontrol.net/news/news-archive/global-surveys-on-rabies-in-progress.html

These three case-studies highlight several key issues that argue for more research on the burden and the costs to humans and to the agricultural/livestock sectors of zoonotic infections. While individual disease studies are useful in quantifying such losses, given that there may be several co-endemic zoonoses, the overall costs of animal-associated infections can be predicted to be much higher, in view of underestimates also from incorrect diagnosis and underreporting.

3.2 Disease-specific issues and burden

3.2.1 Helminths

3.2.1.1 Cysticercosis/taeniasis

Cysticercosis is caused by the tapeworm *Taenia solium* and is transmitted between humans (definitive hosts) and pigs (intermediate hosts). The adult

T. solium causes an intestinal infection, taeniasis in humans, whereas the larval stages cause cysticercosis in both humans and pigs. Owing to conditions related to poverty, such as inadequate sanitation, poor pig management practices, and lack or absence of meat inspection and control, cysticercosis/taeniasis remains an important public health and veterinary problem in many poor countries. In humans, cysticercosis is particularly important as it can lead to a range of neurological disorders and sometimes death. Cysticercosis is also a serious constraint for the nutritional and economic well-being of smallholder farming communities in many countries of Africa, Latin America and Asia as it reduces the market value of pigs and renders pork unsafe to eat. Neurocysticercosis (NCC in humans) occurs when an immature larval stage of the parasite migrates to the brain. It is considered the most common parasitic infection of the human nervous system and the most frequent and preventable cause of epilepsy in the developing world (*35–37*).

In a meta-analysis, lesions of NCC were reported in about 30% of people with epilepsy in endemic countries (*38*). This estimate was similar in both children and adults, which supports reports from southern Africa and India indicating that NCC is a common cause of juvenile epilepsy (*39–46*). In Honduras, a clinical study revealed that 19% of epileptic patients (n=60) had viable intracerebral cysticerci and 65% of them had calcifications compatible with NCC (*37*).

Despite its frequency and severity, little is known about the societal and economical impact of NCC. Initiatives are currently underway to determine the burden of NCC in endemic countries of Africa, Asia and Latin America as well as countries with many imported cases such as the USA (*23, 47*). Cysticercosis is becoming a growing problem in some developed countries because of immigration of infected individuals from endemic areas (*37*).

On the basis of its biological and transmission characteristics, cysticercosis was declared eradicable in 1993 by the International Task Force for Disease Eradication (*48, 49*). But since its eradication is dependent on behavioural changes in endemic populations as well as on implementation of the appropriate biomedical control measures, the disease remains prevalent among impoverished populations. Other factors contributing to the lost opportunity to eradicate the disease are the chronic nature of the infection in humans, the variety of symptoms associated with NCC, the lack of information and awareness about the burden and transmission of the disease, and the lack of field-applicable diagnostic tools for NCC. Despite the 1993 Task Force recommendation, cysticercosis/taeniasis has not been eliminated from any region, no national control programmes are in place, and limited advocacy is being undertaken despite the existence of regional working groups.

WHO included cysticercosis/taeniasis in its Global Plan to Combat Neglected Tropical Diseases 2008–2009 (*50*) and in new initiatives addressing integrated control of neglected zoonotic diseases (*2*, *46*), and in assessing the burden of foodborne diseases (*47–49*). International epilepsy associations are giving increased attention to NCC as a major preventable cause of epilepsy (*50*), and international NCC/cysticercosis working groups have been formed (*51–59*) to facilitate research and control efforts to combat *T. solium* infections.

Two randomized controlled community trials on the effectiveness of strategies to control cysticercosis have been published (*60–61*). In Peru, a randomized community trial in nine villages, split into 12 "treatment units", assessed the effect of combined mass human and pig chemotherapy on the prevalence and incidence rates of porcine cysticercosis (*60*). The descriptive statistics supported some reduction in prevalence and incidence of porcine cysticercosis in the intervention villages as compared with the controls. Another randomized, controlled community trial in 42 villages of northern United Republic of Tanzania aimed at improving pig management through an educational programme. The trial demonstrated that there was a reduction in the incidence of porcine cysticercosis of 49% as measured by circulating antigens in sentinel pigs (*60*). Similarly, a predictive transmission dynamics model indicated that interventions targeting improvement in sanitation and in pig management techniques would be more effective in the long term than treating pigs and/or humans (*61*).

The social consequences of NCC, mostly as a result of epileptic seizures, include stigmatization and incapacitation leading to decreased work productivity (*62–67*). People with epilepsy are often isolated and fail to receive appropriate treatment (*68*, *69*). In west Cameroon it has been estimated that only 27% of people with epilepsy marry and 39% fail to enter any professional activity (*69*), while in Zambia people with epilepsy have poorer employment status, less education, poorer housing and greater food insecurity. Adult females with epilepsy are more likely to deliver their babies at home and are at greater risk of rape (*70*). People with epilepsy are also prone to accidents during seizures, resulting in serious burns from fires, drowning or injury due to automobile accidents, consequences that should also be considered in estimating the burden of NCC (*71*).

Modelling the expected numbers of epilepsy cases associated with NCC revealed that between 2.8 and 20.4 DALYs per thousand persons were lost per year, which was a higher estimate than for some other NTDs (*72*). The DALYs associated with NCC are now being calculated through a systematic review of the literature by a WHO-led initiative to estimate the global burden of foodborne diseases (*52–54*).

3.2.1.2 Cystic and alveolar echinococcosis

Echinococcosis (hydatid disease) is caused by cystic stages of cestode tapeworms belonging to the genus *Echinococcus* (family Taeniidae). The adult worms are found in carnivores, especially dogs and foxes. The two species that infect humans are *Echinococcus granulosus* and *E. multilocularis*, which cause cystic echinococcosis (CE, hydatidosis) and alveolar echinococcosis (AE), respectively. Both infections are responsible for substantial morbidity and mortality. Human CE is the most frequent and accounts for around 95% of the estimated 2–3 million global echinococcosis cases. Recent reports indicate that CE and AE are of increasing public health concern and that both can be regarded as emerging or re-emerging diseases (*73*).

Echinococcus granulosus has a worldwide geographical distribution and is found in at least 100 countries. The highest prevalence is reported from parts of Africa (northern and eastern regions), Eurasia (e.g. central Asia, China, the Mediterranean region, Russia) and South America. The actual prevalence can be from sporadic to high, and few countries can be regarded as being free of the parasite, apart from island states such as Cyprus, Iceland and New Zealand, where elimination campaigns have been successful. The DALYs associated with human CE were recently estimated to be more than for onchocerciasis and similar to African trypanosomiasis (*14*). The socioeconomic impact of CE has not been well researched.

Ingestion of material contaminated with dog faeces containing *E. granulosus* eggs results in the development in humans, or other intermediate hosts, of unilocular fluid-filled bladders – hydatid cysts – mainly in the liver and lungs but also in other organs. Cysts are often asymptomatic but as they increase in size over time they act like tumour masses and cause symptoms due to pressure on surrounding tissues. Cysts may rupture resulting in acute anaphylactic shock and death if untreated. Dogs that harbour the adult worms become infected by ingestion of offal containing viable hydatid cysts. The populations, often pastoral communities, at risk of infection usually live in rural areas where surveillance is difficult as the infection is asymptomatic, in both livestock and dogs, and hence not recognized or prioritized by communities or the local veterinary services.

Treatment for CE relies mainly on surgery or percutaneous drainage to relieve the pressure symptoms, although the latter has been problematic because of the risk of spilling cyst fluid and causing anaphylactic shock. Drug treatment with high doses of albendazole alone or in combination with praziquantel is effective and can also be used before surgery to sterilize cysts (*74*). Percutaneous drainage using ultrasound guidance is better than simply puncturing a cyst. However, ultrasound and/or surgical intervention, which is often difficult, may not be available in resource-poor settings.

Echinococcus multilocularis which causes alveolar echinococcosis is found in the northern hemisphere, including central Europe, most of northern and central Eurasia (extending eastwards to Japan) and parts of North America. The median of the total numbers of AE cases in the world has recently been estimated at some 18 000 cases per year; of these 91% are believed to be in China, particularly on the Tibetan plateau (*75*). The authors (*75*) calculated a median global DALY of 666 434 DALYs per annum. This high rate is attributable to the high fatality rate, resulting in many years of life lost. Adult worm infections of *E. multilocularis* are maintained in a wildlife cycle, with foxes being the most important definitive hosts and small rodents (especially microtine voles) acting as intermediate hosts. Human AE is consequently a rarer zoonosis than CE. The disease is regarded as an emerging disease in Europe because of increasing fox populations. Although foxes are the principal reservoir of adult worms, dogs are increasingly being regarded as hosts (*75*).

The cystic form of *E. multilocularis* is a tumour-like infiltrating structure of numerous small vesicles embedded in stroma of connective tissue that develops almost exclusively in the liver (99% of cases), although metastasis to other organs can occur. The parasitic mass usually contains a semisolid matrix rather than fluid and is associated with progressive disease, a poor response to therapy, a high fatality rate and poor prognosis if managed inappropriately. Radical surgery, which has been has been the cornerstone of treatment for AE, is rarely available in resource-poor populations.

Early diagnosis of AE is crucial and results in a reduced rate of unresectable lesions and less need for more radical surgery. Perioperative and long-term adjuvant chemotherapy with albendazole (doses up to 20 mg/kg per day) has been associated with 10-year survival in approximately 80% of cases, compared with less than 25% in historical controls. Albendazole is parasitostatic only against the *E. multilocularis* metacestode. Liver transplantation has been performed on some AE patients.

The definitive diagnosis of most human cases of CE and AE is by imaging methods, such as radiology, ultrasonography, computerized axial tomography (CT) and scanning or magnetic resonance imaging (MRI). Such procedures are not readily available in isolated communities and poor populations. The advent of lower-cost portable ultrasound scanners now enables community-based surveys in rural endemic regions to be undertaken. Immunodiagnosis (detection of anti-*Echinococcus* antibodies in serum) complements the clinical picture, and is useful not only in primary diagnosis but also for the follow-up of patients after surgery or drug treatment.

Preventive measures that have been used to control *Echinococcus* infections include avoidance of contact with dog or fox faeces, hand-washing and improved sanitation, reducing dog or fox populations, treatment of dogs with arecoline hydrobromide or praziquantel, the use of praziquantel-impregnated baits, incineration of infected organs and health education. Highly successful campaigns using these approaches have eliminated the disease from island nations such as Cyprus, Iceland and New Zealand, where control of dogs and offal consumption is more easily monitored and boundaries for importation secure.

However, despite the establishment of control programmes against CE in some countries or regions, *E. granulosus* still has a wide geographical distribution and the parasite continues to be the cause of substantial morbidity and mortality in many parts of the world. Indeed, recent evidence suggests CE is a public health problem of increasing concern, persisting or re-emerging in many areas of the world, causing severe disease and considerable economic loss (*76*).

A similar situation prevails with *E. multilocularis*, as shown by the increasing prevalence of AE, its distribution, which is wider than previously thought, and the fact that the parasite can readily spread from endemic to non-endemic areas. The greater pathogenicity, difficulty of treatment and higher mortality risk of AE have led to intervention trials/programmes for control in a number of endemic areas. However, effective methods for control of *E. multilocularis* are not yet available, and this lends support to the argument for more efficient prevention measures and early diagnosis of AE.

In some areas, notably western China, both human AE and CE are co-endemic, and combined control of these *Echinococcus* species may be warranted. Guidelines should be developed for consideration of definitions for control of CE so as to determine what levels of reduction in sheep, dog and human infections will have a significant impact. Chemotherapy has reduced the need for invasive surgical management of CE and AE, but there is a need for new advances in the prevention and control of both diseases.

3.2.1.3 **Zoonotic Asian schistosomiasis**

Asian schistosomiasis is caused by the trematodes *Schistosoma japonicum* and *Schistosoma mekongi*. *S. mekongi* infects humans in Cambodia and the southern tip of the Lao People's Democratic Republic, while *S. japonicum* infections are endemic in China, in parts of Indonesia and in the Philippines. Even though 40 mammalian species have been shown to harbour *S. japonicum* (*77*), only 10 are considered to contribute significantly to human infection (*78–80*). *S. japonicum* and *S. mekongi* are transmitted through contact with fresh water that contains free-swimming larval forms called cercariae released from snails, which are the intermediate hosts. Cercariae penetrate the skin of the mammalian hosts and develop into adult worms. Water buffalo, cattle, rodents, dogs, sheep and pigs act as reservoirs for transmission of *S. japonicum* and dogs and pigs are the main reservoirs for *S. mekongi*.

Male and female worms migrate to the hepatic portal system where they mature, pair up and move downstream. The worm pairs reach mucosal branches of the inferior mesenteric and superior haemorrhoidal veins and the females then begin egg production. The process of migration and maturation takes 4–5 weeks. Eggs pass through the intestinal wall and are discharged in the faeces into freshwater. The miracidia are explosively liberated from the eggs while still encapsulated within their sub-shell envelopes and infect receptive *Oncomelania hupensis* (*S. japonicum*) or *Neotricula aperta* (*S. mekongi*) snails.

In humans, *S. japonicum* is associated with liver disease, splenomegaly and bloody diarrhoea, malnutrition, anaemia and reduced cognition (*81*). In a recent review of the literature, the disability weights associated with *S. japonicum* were found to be between 7 and 46 times larger than those used in the latest global burden of disease estimates (*82*).

The contribution of different animal species to infection of humans may vary in different endemic areas. In China, studies support a major contribution of cattle and water buffalo in the transmission of *S. japonicum* to humans (*81*). This is in contrast to the Philippines, where studies in Samar Province found an association between the intensity of infection in dogs and cats and infection in humans (*83*). However, using a polymerase chain reaction (PCR)-based diagnostic method (*84*), the prevalence of *S. japonicum* in water buffalo (carabao) was as high as 60% in some communities (*84*). Hence the importance of their role in disease transmission in the Philippines needs to be clarified.

A mass treatment approach with praziquantel has proved effective in some areas of China and eliminated *S. mekongi* in Cambodia (*85*). However, it remains less effective in other schistosomiasis-endemic provinces (*86*). In both China and the Philippines, infection in the mammalian reservoir hosts has prevented the possible elimination of schistosomiasis (*87*). Also, some communities are reluctant to accept the mass distribution of praziquantel (*88*).

A pilot study for integrated control of schistosomiasis has recently been undertaken in China. The study involved a multi-pronged approach of removing bovines from snail-infested grasslands, providing farmers with mechanized farm equipment, improving sanitation by supplying tap water and building lavatories and latrines, providing boats with containers for faeces disposal, and implementing an intensive health education programme (*89*). This comprehensive control strategy based on interventions to reduce the rate of transmission of *S. japonicum* infection from cattle and humans to snails has been highly effective. As a result the Chinese government has adopted the interventions used in the study as the national strategy for the control of schistosomiasis. However, replacement of bovines with machinery may not be feasible in many schistosomiasis-endemic areas, such as lakes/marshlands or mountainous regions because of the difficult terrain. The cost of large-scale implementation could prove to be prohibitive.

Additional challenges to elimination include the limited accuracy of field diagnosis using the Kato-Katz technique, the poor compliance of some populations with mass chemotherapy (*88*), the need for sustained, integrated control efforts (*90*), and acceptance of transmission-blocking vaccines in buffalo and other reservoir hosts when they become available for future deployment (*91*). Mathematical modelling has shown that integrated control strategies (including combinations of treatment, bovine vaccination, improved sanitation and reduced water contact) are, indeed, effective for short- and long-term control of Asian schistosomiasis (*81*).

There are other important factors that have yet to be given adequate attention for the control of Asian schistosomiasis. For example, the completion of the Three Gorges Dam in southern China has been predicted to increase transmission of *S. japonicum* (*81*). To reduce the impact of this massive infrastructural project, planners and managers should integrate health impact assessments and examine how families and communities cope with the social and economic changes and health risks resulting from such a project (*92*). An economic analysis has been conducted to evaluate the cost–effectiveness of the 10-year programme that eliminated *S. mekongi* and concluded that for each dollar invested the benefit was over 3 dollars (*93*).

3.2.1.4 Foodborne trematodiases

Foodborne trematodiases (FBTs) are an emerging public health problem. An estimated 750 million people are at risk of acquiring these infections (*94*). The FBTs of public health importance are the liver flukes (*Clonorchis sinensis*, *Fasciola gigantica*, *Fasciola hepatica*, *Opisthorchis felineus*, and *Opisthorchis viverrini*), lung flukes (*Paragonimus* spp.) and intestinal flukes (e.g. *Echinostoma* spp., *Fasciolopsis buski* and the heterophyids). Adult flukes are hermaphroditic and have life-cycles that follow the typical trematode pattern, involving a mollusc intermediate host from which cercariae are released and either encyst on grass or water plants (*F. hepatica*, *F. gigantica*, *F. buski*), penetrate the skin of a secondary intermediate fish host and encyst in the muscles of fish (*C. sinensis*, *O. viverrini*, *Echinostoma* spp.), in crustaceans (e.g. *Paragonimus* spp.) or in frogs, snails and tadpoles (*Echinostoma* spp.). Definitive hosts become infected by eating raw, pickled or insufficiently cooked aquatic products harbouring metacercariae or drinking contaminated water. After ingestion of the metacercariae, excystation of the metacercariae occurs in the stomach and the released juvenile worm migrates to the target organ.

Opisthorchis viverrini is considered a Group I carcinogen (known to be carcinogenic in humans) and long-term infection can lead to cholangiocarcinoma – cancer of the bile ducts. The link between fluke infection and cholangiocarcinoma is less robust for *Clonorchis* spp, but may nonetheless be real (*95*). Detection of eggs in faeces (intestinal flukes, liver flukes and lung flukes) and sputum (lung flukes) is the method of diagnosis of foodborne trematode infections in epidemiological surveys and for the monitoring of control interventions. Serology and ultrasound provide indirect evidence of infection. PCR techniques have been recently introduced to diagnose *Opisthorchis* infections (*95, 96*). Praziquantel exhibits a broad spectrum of activity against trematodes and has an excellent safety profile. Hence it is the drug of choice for clonorchiasis, opisthorchiasis, paragonimiasis and intestinal fluke infections (*94*).

Sheep, goats and cattle are the predominant animal reservoirs of *Fasciola*. In humans, diagnosis of fascioliasis is by finding the eggs in stools, but may be complemented by immunological detection of anti-*F. hepatica* antibodies in sera. Other non-invasive diagnostic techniques are radiology, radioisotope scanning, ultrasound, CT scanning and MRI (*97*). Triclabendazole (10–12 mg/kg) is the drug of choice in human fascioliasis: praziquantel has no effect on *Fasciola* (*92*). Prevention is possible by controlling ingestion of watercress and other metacercariae-carrying aquatic plants consumed by humans, but requires behavioral change in dietary habits (*97*). Triclabendazole has been donated to WHO for the control of fascioliasis by Novartis and is currently being used in mass chemotherapy in Bolivia and Peru.

The increasing impact of FBT infections on human health and productivity is attributed to the rapid development of aquaculture, especially in Asia (*98*). Sixteen per cent of the world's protein consumption and around one quarter of animal protein needs in Asia are met by aquaculture products from backyard ponds, small farms or from industrial settings. In 1999, FAO reported that the global output of aquatic products was 42.77 million tonnes and was valued at US$ 47.86 billion. Ninety per cent of these products are harvested in Asia, of which one-third are from China. Over two-thirds of the world's aquaculture occurs in fresh water, mostly in Asia where FBTs are endemic (*99*). Populations residing near bodies of fresh water, especially in south-east Asia and the Western Pacific region, are at the greatest risk of FBT diseases (*100*). One study demonstrated the increase over a period of only one year in *C. sinensis* infection in farmed fish of some 11% in the Red River Delta in Viet Nam (*98*). The authors recommend that aquaculture management programmes should address the FBT problem, given that young fish are already infected when introduced into grow-out systems.

FBT infections are becoming increasingly common in urban areas as a result of improvements in transportation, marketing and distribution of freshwater fish, crustaceans and edible water plants and because of the embedded practice in many Asian cultures of eating raw freshwater-derived food. The demand for aquaculture-derived products is predicted to increase within the next two decades owing to overfishing of wild fish, rising incomes, increasing population and global demand for high-value protein (*94*).

Despite the availability of interventions for control and treatment of FBT infections, many people dependent on freshwater resources continue to suffer from FBT diseases. Poverty, poor access to health services, lack of education, inadequate health and sanitation facilities, use of human and animal excreta/ wastes as fish feeds, cultural beliefs, and practices concerning the consumption of raw freshwater products are the factors that predispose communities to FBT infections. This situation is aggravated by limited national and local policies, regulations and health services. The participation of social scientists in FBT control programmes is essential to address the importance of health education in guiding people's food habits and to develop appropriate communication and education strategies for behaviour modification.

3.2.2 Protozoan infections

3.2.2.1 Toxoplasmosis

Toxoplasma gondii is an obligate intracellular parasite. Felines are the definitive hosts and act as a reservoir for the parasite. Human infections are acquired by ingestion of cysts (bradyzoites) in infected raw meat or following consumption of food contaminated with sporulated oocysts from cat faeces. Human-to-human transmission is through congenital infection acquired via the transplacental route and can result in premature birth, eye damage and blindness, brain damage causing microcephaly and mental retardation, hydrocephaly, seizures or hepatosplenomegaly. Infection is usually asymptomatic with a low incidence of overt disease. It presents as an acute mononucleosis-like syndrome, chorioretinitis or chronic abortion in women. Of HIV-seropositive patients, 40% develop central nervous system (CNS) toxoplasmosis with focal abscesses primarily located in the brain. Neurological imaging (CT or MRI) is required for diagnosis of CNS toxoplasmosis, but early treatment and prophylaxis have been shown to be effective in diagnosed cases.

Toxoplasmosis has a worldwide distribution, with an estimated one third of the entire global population infected. The US Centers for Disease Control and Prevention estimates that more than 60 million people are infected with the parasite in the USA alone, the vast majority of whom are asymptomatic. In the USA, between 500 and 5000 infants are estimated to be infected annually through the congenital route. Toxoplasmosis is considered to be the third leading cause of death attributable to foodborne illness globally. The burden of toxoplasmosis is borne disproportionately by poor communities in which food safety is inadequate. Limited access to routine prenatal evaluation for toxoplasmosis, which has proved to be effective in preventing neonatal neurological and ocular damage, adds to the burden (*101*). The prevalence of toxoplasmosis is strongly correlated with socioeconomic status (*102*) and environmental humidity. However, the proportion of human infections that derive from these different routes of transmission is not known. Transplantation of infected organs can also result in fatal infection as a consequence of immunosuppressive treatment.

3.2.2.2 Cryptosporidiosis

Awareness of *Cryptosporidium* as a human pathogen began in the early period of the AIDS epidemic, when severe persisting watery diarrhoea was identified as a common concomitant of HIV infection in developed and developing countries (*103*). There are now 18 species and 40 genotypes of *Cryptosporidium* recognized, with nine species and two genotypes associated with human infection (*104*). These species and genotypes are adapted to different hosts, and each species has a variable host range. *Cryptosporidium hominis* is generally non-zoonotic, i.e. humans acquire infection from other humans, whereas the primary source of *C. parvum* infection in humans is zoonotic. Ruminants are the host species, primarily young bovines, although the parasite can subsequently be directly propagated within a human community. Consequently, data from developed countries show that *C. parvum* is most commonly isolated from sporadic human cases originating in rural areas, whereas *C. hominis* predominates in urban settings (*105*, *106*). The best evidence for the zoonotic transmission of *C. parvum* comes from studies of infections among children at a farm day camp, middle- and high-school students in an educational farm programme, and veterinary students in contact with infected bovines (*107–110*).

The advent of highly active antiretroviral therapy (HAART) for HIV patients and the ability to repair immune deficiencies has changed outcomes in such patients (*111*). However, as more investigators searched for evidence of *Cryptosporidium* infection in non-AIDS patients with diarrhoea, it became clear that many self-limited episodes occur in individuals with a normal immune system, especially young children (*112*). The remarkably low infectious dose, and the importance of person-to-person direct transmission has been documented in a human volunteer study (*113*), which found that 18 of 29 normal *Cryptosporidium*-seronegative human adult volunteers became infected and excreted the organism after ingestion of a mean infective dose of just 132 *C. parvum* oocysts. Of these 18 volunteers, 11 were symptomatic and 7 developed diarrhoea. All participants recovered with a mean duration of symptoms of 74 hours (*108*). The difference between self-limited diarrhoea in immunocompetent individuals and chronic diarrhoea in AIDS patients is highlighted by the outcome of a massive waterborne outbreak of infection in Milwaukee, Wisconsin, USA in 1993, when an estimated 403,000 individuals were infected (*114*). When the infection was stratified by HIV status, it was clear that HIV-positive individuals experienced longer-lasting and more severe symptoms and they were more likely to be hospitalized (*115*). Out of 209 children with diarrhoea who had appropriate stool examinations during the outbreak, 49 (23%) were confirmed to be infected with *Cryptosporidium*. These children were more likely to have had an underlying disease that altered their immune status, and the clinical illness was more prolonged and associated with weight loss and abdominal cramps compared with *Cryptosporidium*-negative children. Epidemiological data from both adults and children strongly suggest that effective HAART therapy in AIDS patients ameliorates clinical cryptosporidiosis as host immunocompetence is restored (*116*). The estimated cost of the illnesses associated with the Milwaukee outbreak was over US$ 96 million, including US$ 31.7 million in medical costs and US$ 64.6 million in productivity losses (*117*). The implications of these data for the setting in developing countries are obvious: 1) the size of the ruminant host population for *C. parvum*; 2) the close interactions between people and livestock in rural settings, and the small infectious dose; 3) the consequences of oocyst contamination of drinking-water; 4) the susceptibility of young or immunocompromised individuals; 5) the relevance of common risk reduction strategies for this and other zoonotic and marginalized infections through improved water safety and hygienic practices.

In the USA, the most recent period of surveillance indicates a confirmed infection rate of approximately 4/100 000 person-years (*118*). Infants and children in group settings in which personal hygiene is difficult to maintain are at higher risk of infection through direct person-to-person or person-to-food/water-to-person transmission. In developing countries, the prevalence is particularly high in children aged 6–36 months, associated with both malnutrition and/or HIV infection (*119*). In Guinea-Bissau, West Africa, nearly 8% of diarrhoeal stools from children were positive for *Cryptosporidium* (*120*) and, by the age of two, 45% of children had been infected (*121*). In such settings, infection is commonly associated with persistent diarrhoea, and multiple species of the parasite may be involved, although the vast majority of infections are due to *C. hominis* (87%) and *C. parvum* (9%) (*122*). Diarrhoeal stools from 848 children under 5 years of age in urban and rural hospital settings in Malawi were examined for *Cryptosporidium* oocysts (123). Of the 50 oocyst-positive samples, 43 could be amplified by PCR restriction fragment length polymorphism. On the basis of this analysis, samples from children in rural areas showed a wider species range than samples from children in urban areas, suggesting the importance of zoonotic transmission in rural settings.

Diagnosis of cryptosporidiosis, especially in developing countries, depends primarily on simple differential staining techniques and microscopy, although sensitive and specific immunological and nucleic acid-based diagnostics are available but are costly (*124*). An advantage of microscopy for *Cryptosporidium* is that other infections (e.g. helminth ova) can also be detected during microscopic examination. On the other hand, with a single specimen examined by microscopy it is easy to miss the diagnosis, since the number of oocysts excreted can vary during the course of symptomatic infection and at times may be below the detectable limits (*125*). There is little doubt that new sensitive, specific and inexpensive tests would be useful, particularly if they could distinguish between *C. hominis* and *C. parvum*, thus suggesting likely transmission routes to investigate.

Prevention and treatment of cryptosporidiosis are problematic. Maintaining personal hygiene for infants and toddlers is difficult. Infected individuals may continue to pass oocysts for several weeks after a clinical infection (*125*). Similarly, it can be difficult to prevent contamination of water sources by animals. Drug treatment has been disappointing (*126*). The one drug licensed to treat cryptosporidiosis in non-immunocompromised individuals, nitazoxanide, may shorten the course and duration of excretion of oocysts. However, it is of limited value in self-limiting infection in immunocompetent individuals and less effective in chronic infection in the immunocompromised. Indeed, a controlled trial in children with AIDS in Zambia demonstrated no efficacy of the drug, and the authors concluded that the drug could not be recommended for treatment of cryptosporidiosis in Zambian children with AIDS (*129*).

There are economic consequences of *Cryptosporidium* infection in cattle, primarily related to the costs of care of animals with diarrhoea and dehydration, slower growth, and some associated mortality (*128*). Although a number of investigators believe there is a significant economic cost of cryptosporidiosis in calves (*129*), it is difficult to find quantitative data, especially in developing country settings. Without these data, strategies to prevent or treat bovine infections may be less appealing to producers, particularly small-scale farms, than a strategy to prevent or mitigate infection in humans. This is primarily through better agricultural practices to limit spread of oocysts in water or food crops grown near cattle or dairy herds, or through effective filtration of drinking-water.

3.2.3 Bacterial infections

3.2.3.1 Brucellosis

Brucellosis is a bacterial zoonosis, caused by intracellular bacteria of the genus *Brucella* (*130*). The genus includes six species producing disease in terrestrial animals, with *Brucella melitensis*, *Brucella abortus* and *Brucella suis* being the most pathogenic species. These bacteria infect a variety of domestic livestock such as goats, cattle, camels, sheep and pigs. *Brucella* is a major cause of zoonotic infections and therefore is of serious public health importance, particularly in low-income countries where intervention strategies are almost non-existent (*130*). Brucella infections are also widespread in wild mammals, including marine mammals (*131*). Thus, the impact and distribution of this disease in wild animal populations deserves attention. In the animal primary host, brucellosis induces abortions and genital infections, which are the major sources of economic losses.

Humans are usually infected through consumption of non-pasteurized dairy products and close-contact manipulation of infected animals. Human brucellosis is a severely debilitating disease characterized by persistent waves of fever (and therefore known as undulant fever) and a suite of nonspecific manifestations such as headache, malaise, back pain, myalgia and generalized aches. Splenomegaly, hepatomegaly, coughing and pleuritic chest pain are sometimes seen (*132*). Gastrointestinal symptoms, including anorexia, nausea, vomiting, diarrhoea and constipation, occur frequently in adults but less often in children. If not treated, the infection can progress to granulomatous hepatitis, uveitis, meningitis, endocarditis or other manifestations. The nonspecific clinical presentation of *Brucella* infections results in widespread misdiagnosis and underreporting of the condition, particularly in malaria-endemic areas, where fevers are often assumed to be malaria (*133*, *134*). These problems are compounded by lack of sufficient knowledge about the disease among health staff (*135*), the variable performance of serological diagnostic tests (*136*), and delays in health-seeking behaviour (*137*).

It is likely that the incidence of human disease varies considerably in different communities, in line with the wide geographical variation in livestock seroprevalence patterns in different agro-ecological settings (*138*). However, there is no doubt that, in many areas, the disease burden is likely to be substantial. Results from a population-based study in rural areas of the United Republic of Tanzania indicated that 13% of people sampled in pastoral communities were seropositive, with 43% of seropositive individuals showing at least two clinical symptoms consistent with brucellosis (*139*). Although brucellosis has been eliminated from several countries, largely as a result of test-and-slaughter and vaccination programmes in livestock populations, the disease remains widespread and poses public health threats throughout Africa, South America, Asia and parts of Europe.

3.2.3.2 Enteric infections

Enteric infections are among the most common afflictions of humans. They contribute to a high proportion of deaths in low- and middle-income countries in all regions of the world (Figures 2 and 3). Most individuals will have an episode of watery diarrhoea (defined as three or more liquid non-bloody stools per day for an individual older than 3 months and five or more liquid stools for a breastfeeding infant under 3 months of age) at least once or, more likely, several times a year. Complicating etiological diagnosis is the fact that there are multiple bacterial and viral pathogens, protozoa (especially *Cryptosporidium hominis* or *parvum*, *Giardia intestinalis* and *Balantidium coli*), and intestinal helminths that also cause occasional diarrhoea in humans. The vast majority of these episodes are mild, self-limiting and more a nuisance than a significant illness. In developing countries it is quite different, as the lack of safe water and effective sanitation and household hygiene contribute to multiple episodes of more severe illness, especially in young children. Watery diarrhoea, associated with losses of 10% or more of body water and electrolytes, results in severe dehydration, hypotension and life-threatening circulatory collapse. *Vibrio cholerae* and enterotoxigenic or enteropathogenic *Escherichia coli* (ETEC or EPEC) are frequent causes of dehydrating diarrhoea in children under 5 years, while cholera and ETEC are major pathogens in those older than 5, including adults (*140*). In young children, some 5–10% of watery diarrhoea episodes persist beyond 14 days. These illnesses are associated with significant malabsorption and malnutrition, are disproportionately associated with a fatal outcome, and require particular attention to nutritional interventions, and for these reasons should be separately classified as persistent diarrhoea (*141*).

In addition to dehydrating diarrhoea and persistent diarrhoea, however, other enteric pathogens exhibit distinctive pathogenic mechanisms resulting in marked inflammatory responses in the intestinal mucosa. This results in mucosal ulcerations due to intestinal epithelial cell death which leads to bloody diarrhoea or dysentery. The latter is a more clinically severe syndrome defined by the triad of a characteristic small-volume bloody stool with leukocytes and mucus, abdominal cramps, and tenesmus, a worsening of abdominal symptoms with the urge to pass stools. The commonest cause of inflammatory diarrhoea or dysentery is the genus *Shigella*, the cause of shigellosis or bacillary dysentery. These bacteria invade the mucosa and initiate pro-inflammatory cytokine responses with profound metabolic effects. These include anorexia and reduced intake of food, losses of carbohydrate stores, minerals and micronutrients, protein-losing enteropathy due to losses of serum proteins across the damaged mucosa into the gut lumen, catabolism of muscle protein, and changes in priorities for hepatic protein synthesis from albumin to acute-phase proteins modulating host defence responses (*142*). These effects last far beyond the period of acute clinical illness, and account for ongoing loss of lean body mass during convalescence (*143*). When additional infections of any nature (enteric, respiratory or systemic viral or bacterial infections) occur in rapid succession (especially when accompanied by fever, which exacerbates catabolic losses) and before nutritional deficits can be restored, a progressive decline in nutritional status is initiated, leading ultimately to severe protein-energy malnutrition. Without appropriate nutritional interventions, death is a frequent outcome. Unfortunately, this is a common scenario among children under 5 years of age in developing countries, as one infection follows another, each resulting in some loss of nutrient stores, without the possibility to correct the loss before the next infection occurs (*144*). For this reason malnutrition is associated with more than half of childhood deaths, and is a major risk factor even when a specific terminal illness is identified (*57*). Because enteric infections are such important contributors to progressive nutritional decline, they are frequent antecedent causes of death, regardless of the terminal event.

The delayed effects of enteric diseases, especially inflammatory diarrhoea, can easily be underestimated in assigning causes of death, and therefore their impact is generally far greater than usually believed. Recent studies of inpatient deaths indicate that use of standard anthropometric methods to assess overall nutritional status underestimates the effect of malnutrition (*145*). Such studies show that the attributable fractional risk of death due to malnutrition exceeds 50%. The original characterization of the interaction of malnutrition and infectious diseases as synergistic (*146*) remains an operationally valid way to consider the relationship. Unfortunately, prospects are not encouraging, since population increase in many developing countries continues unabated, and the effects of climate change and severe weather events are becoming more common, with potential serious effects on soil quality, food supply and nutritional status. All this undermines efforts to diminish poverty and improve nutrition and general health status. Food insecurity is a major ongoing global crisis.

Current estimates suggest that overall mortality due to all enteric infections in infants and children under 5 years of age is around 1.9 million deaths per year (*147*), second only to acute pneumonia as a cause of death among this age group. This estimate is derived from analysis of published reports, mostly from facility-based studies, rather than the community. The proportion of under-5 deaths due to diarrhoeal disease is highest in the South-East Asia and Africa Regions of WHO (Figures 2 and 3).

Figure 2
Distribution of deaths due to diarrhoea in low- and middle-income countries in five WHO regions

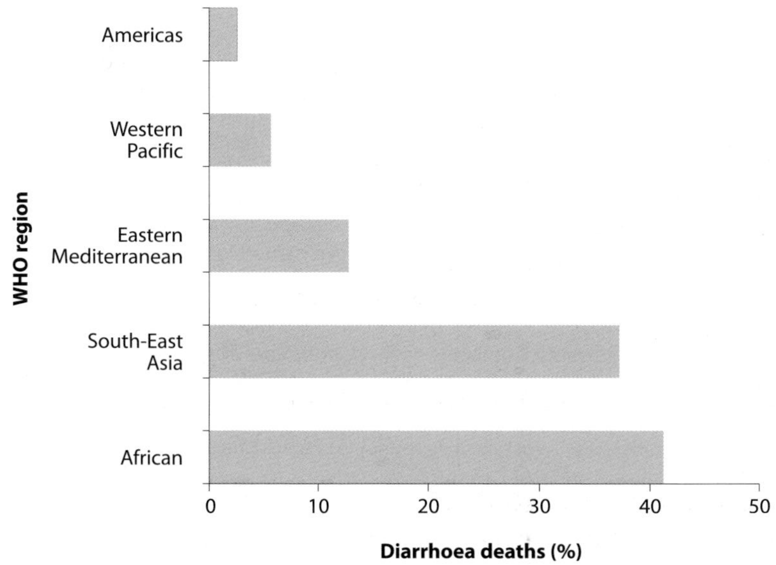

Figure 3
Worldwide distribution of deaths caused by diarrhea in children under 5 years of age in 2000 (*148*)

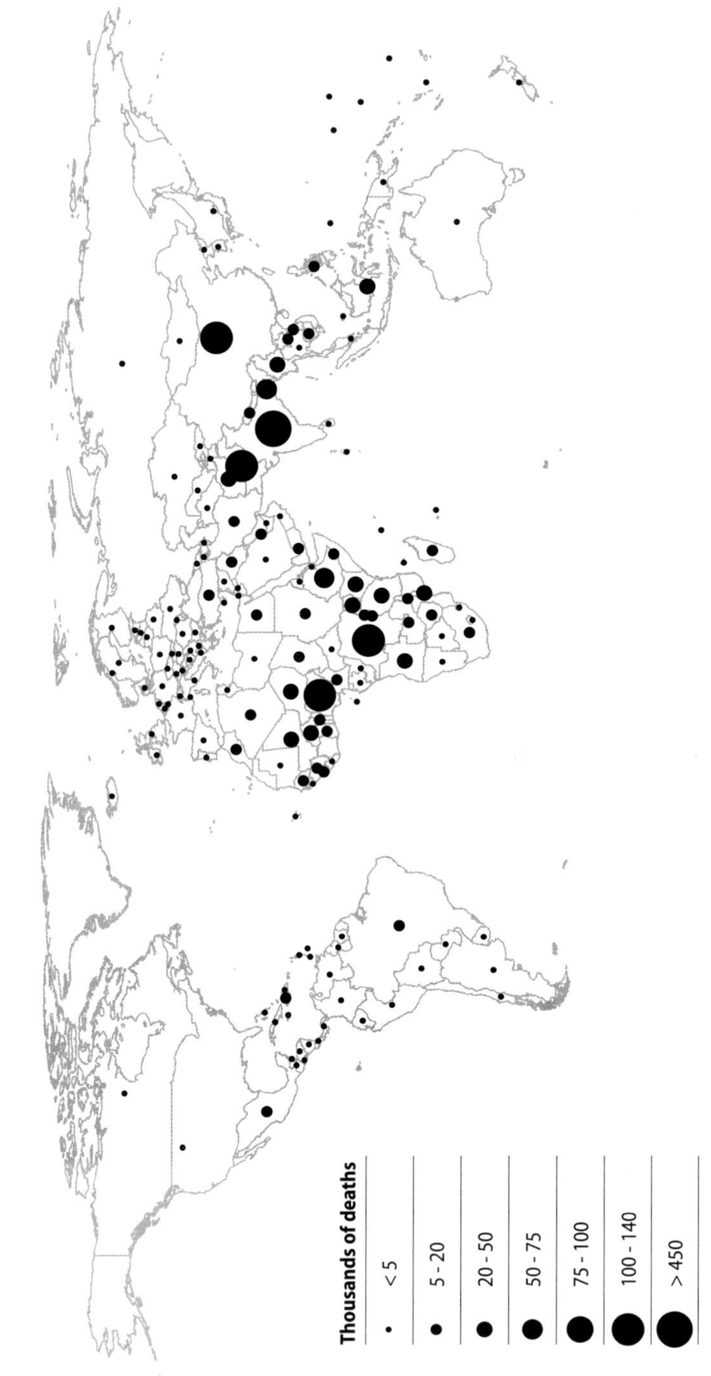

The reports on which these analyses are based, in general, provide no specific information on the prevalence of watery, inflammatory or persistent diarrhoea, and little if any information on the specific etiological causes. As many as 25% of these deaths are thought to be due to rotavirus infection, which occurs primarily in infants under 2 years of age, who are highly vulnerable to rapid dehydration. A considerable but uncertain proportion of the remainder are likely to be due to *Shigella* infection, which is not particularly mitigated by effective rehydration interventions. A previous estimate of 1.1 million deaths/year due to *Shigella* species (*149*) is now considered to be excessive, but no better or more recent estimates are available. Persistent diarrhoea is a distinctive syndrome, may occur in 5–15% of episodes in vulnerable populations, and is associated with ongoing malabsorption and malnutrition rather than rapid dehydration. Persistent diarrhoea has a higher case-fatality rate than acute watery or inflammatory diarrhoea, and may account for as much as 30–50% of diarrhoeal disease deaths (*141*).

Nonetheless, estimated mortality due to enteric infections in young children has progressively decreased over the past 30 years. During this time the number of children under 5 at risk in the world has increased several-fold (*140*). This is a remarkable achievement, much of which can be attributed to the success of oral rehydration to correct severe dehydration, to recognition of persistent diarrhoea as a problem, to improvements in nutritional status through programmes for nutritional rehabilitation and micronutrient supplements, and to a lesser extent to the use of antibiotics to treat bloody diarrhoea and dysentery.

There are several caveats in interpreting these data. Firstly, there is only limited information on the prevalence of inflammatory diarrhoea and dysentery. Secondly, (in contrast to the ongoing effectiveness of oral rehydration therapy), sustaining the impact of antibiotics for bloody diarrhoea and dysentery is a serious concern. This is due to the continuing selection and spread of bacterial resistance to the readily available, oral, safe and effective drugs. Thirdly, nutritional status and access to care have improved in some parts of the developing world and they are likely to be favourably affecting outcomes of diarrhoeal disease. Fourthly, increasing numbers of HIV/AIDS patients are being treated with antiretroviral therapy, which will improve the host immune response to infections and reduce susceptibility to infections for which treatment is of limited benefit, e.g. cryptosporidiosis. These observations suggest that the causes and responses to enteric diseases to further reduce the mortality toll are likely to be changing over time. Finally, there has been no reduction in the incidence of diarrhoea in children under 5 for the past 30 years, and so any deterioration in health systems, environmental sanitation or access to safe water, or treatment failures due to antimicrobial drug resistance, may reverse the current overall favourable trends.

From another perspective, diarrhoeal diseases are estimated to be responsible for 72.8 million DALYs (4.8% of all DALYs) among all ages and all regions of the world, second only to respiratory diseases as a source of global DALYs (*150–154*). The distribution of these DALYs, however, is highly related to economic status. Among low-income countries, diarrhoeal diseases accounted for 59.2 million DALYs, whereas there were just over 400 000 DALYs in high-income countries, and only some 14 000 deaths. It is much more difficult to assess the incidence of enteric infections. Such calculations are subject to great variation depending on: 1) the method used and the quality of data collection; 2) the representative nature of the population studied (they are likely to over-sample health facilities rather than the community and underestimate cases of mild/moderate diarrhoea); 3) the infrastructure for the supply of clean water, sanitary disposal of faeces and safe storage of food; 4) the relative prevalence of specific agents and whether or not they are affected by chlorination or water filtration; 5) low-inoculum pathogens that can be readily transmitted by person-to-person contact.

Mortality rates are dependent on the frequency of all infections, as well as on the availability of health-care facilities and access to treatment, including rehydration, antibiotics and nutritional rehabilitation services. The difference between high- and low-income countries is greatest for mortality and least for incidence, with severe illness and hospitalization somewhere in between. Some enteric pathogens, such as *Vibrio cholerae* O1 or O139 and *Shigella dysenteriae* Type 1, also have epidemic potential, when the impact on older children and adults is increased. Global trends for cholera tracked by WHO show a steady increase in cholera reporting in recent years (*155*). Thus during the period 2004–2008 a cumulative total of 838 315 cases were reported to WHO, which is a 24% increase over the 676 651 cases reported during the period 2000–2004. There was a concomitant 27.5% increase in cholera deaths.

Cholera is still underreported in some regions, particularly in south-east and central Asia, where inconsistencies in case definitions and lack of a standard vocabulary hinder case identification. Some countries report only laboratory-confirmed infections, and so there are large numbers of cases consistent with the WHO standard case definition that, as a result, go unreported. Notification of cholera also does not include cases labelled as acute watery diarrhoea in Africa and central and south-east Asia, for which there are many causes and where microbiological laboratory support is commonly unavailable. An unknown but substantial proportion of the 500 000–700 000 episodes labelled acute watery diarrhoea annually are certainly due to *V. cholerae*. This is supported by a recent study from India, which substantiates the gross underreporting of cholera due to incomplete and/or inadequate data collection (*156*). Over 220 000 cases were identified by the authors over a 10 year period, which contrasts with the nearly 38 000 cases reported to WHO during the same time period. In the case of *S. dysenteriae* Type 1, carefully collected data from Bangladesh show that *S. dysenteriae* Type 1 has virtually disappeared over the past 10 years (Figure 4).

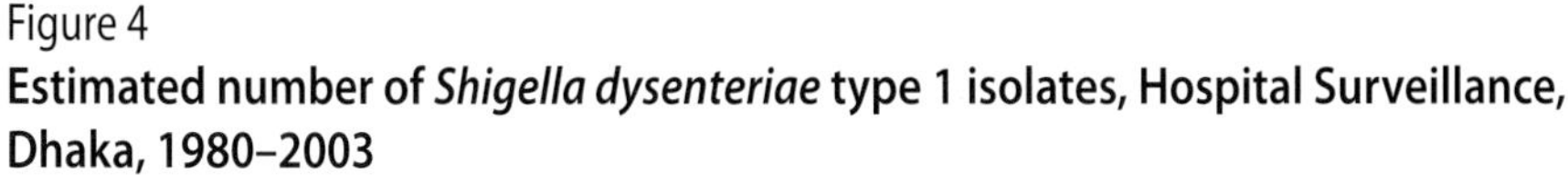

Figure 4
Estimated number of *Shigella dysenteriae* type 1 isolates, Hospital Surveillance, Dhaka, 1980–2003

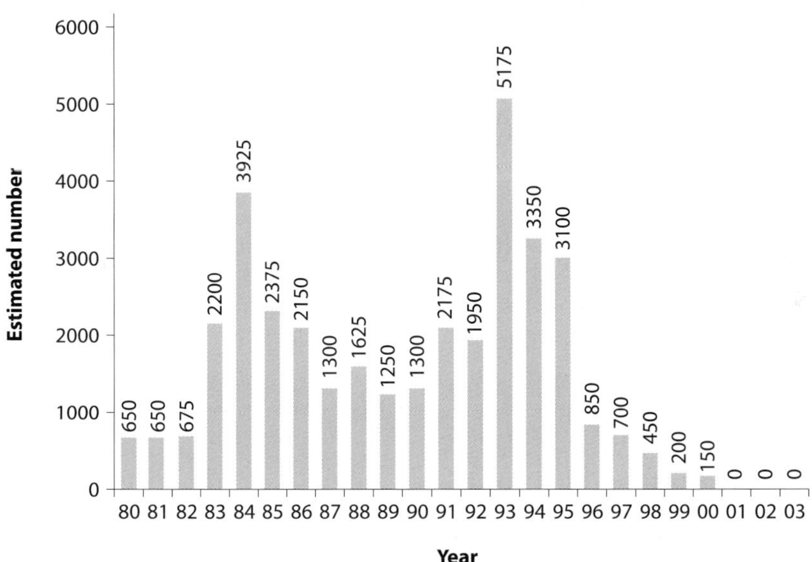

Permission by icddr,b
(From Figure 1: Estimated number of *S. Dysenteriae* type 1 isolates, Hospital Surveillance, Dhaka, 1980-2003 in "Increasing Antibiotic Resistance of *Shigella* species". Health and Science Bulletin Vol 2, No 1, March 2004)

Similar findings have been reported from Africa, where surveillance is limited to a small number of facilities with diagnostic capabilities (*157*). Whether or not this trend will be sustained cannot be predicted, in part because this organism has remained in the background for long periods in the past before suddenly reappearing in explosive and devastating epidemics.

Dehydrating watery diarrhoea outbreaks (e.g. cholera, ETEC) and dysentery (e.g. *S. dysenteriae* Type 1) are particular problems in situations of complex humanitarian disasters and emergencies, whether due to war and violence or to natural disasters.

Following the devastating earthquake in January 2010 in Haiti, cholera was reported in October 2010. By the end of 2011, over half a million cases had occurred, with over 7000 deaths. Currently, some 200 cases a day are being reported during the dry season, rising 5-fold during the wet season (*206*). Refugees from either war and violence or natural disasters are typically gathered in temporary camps, which are initially chaotic and lack adequate clean water or facilities for personal hygiene and sanitary disposal of human faeces, or access to appropriate medical care. Children and even adults are highly susceptible to enteric infections under these circumstances, and history has documented waves of watery diarrhoea followed by dysentery and malnutrition, with case-fatality rates as high as 9% (*158*). In some instances enteric infections have been the cause of more than 40% of the reported deaths, over 80% of which have occurred in children under 2, mostly due to cholera and *Shigella* infection (*159*).

While cholera and dysentery have historically been associated with military campaigns (*160*) and mass migrations, such as the annual pilgrimage to Mecca (*161, 162*), attention to safe water supplies and disposal of faeces by the Kingdom of Saudi Arabia has reduced the frequency of outbreaks in recent years, although sporadic cases still occur (*163*). However, pilgrims returning home can still initiate secondary cholera outbreaks where conditions are conducive to waterborne spread. Even developed countries continue to report sporadic cases of cholera acquired, in the case of the USA, through ingestion of contaminated raw shellfish harvested from the Gulf of Mexico where *V. cholerae* O1 lives in its natural coastal water habitat. Outbreak spread is effectively prevented by access to safe chlorinated water sources and infrastructure for the sanitary disposal of faeces.

Many of the pathogens involved in zoonotic diarrhoeal disease in humans colonize the animal host but do not result in disease. Non-typhoidal *Salmonella*, *E. coli* O157:H7, *Campylobacter jejuni* and *Cryptosporidium parvum* are examples. Livestock and poultry populations can frequently be infected but are uncommonly affected. However, foodborne illness in the USA has been estimated to cause 76 million new cases per year, resulting in 325 000 hospitalizations and some 5000 deaths (*164*). A recent report (*165*) estimates the cost of these illnesses at US$ 152 billion per year, not including the costs to industry due to recalls of tainted foods or the impact of consumer avoidance of consumption of suspect foods. The global cost of emerging epidemic infections, including SARS, and H5N1 and H1N1 influenza virus, has been estimated to total around US$ 200 million over the past decade in initiating targeted surveillance, culling animals to stop spread of infection, and trade- and tourism-related losses (*166*).

3.2.3.3 Bovine tuberculosis

The disease burden of zoonotic tuberculosis (caused by *Mycobacterium bovis*) remains largely unknown, despite widespread recognition of its potential to contribute to the human tuberculosis epidemic, particularly in the era of HIV/AIDS (*167–172*). Problems relate both to laboratory diagnosis, which requires specialized culture facilities that are rarely available in developing countries, and to a lack of awareness among clinicians of the potential for species other than *M. tuberculosis* to cause tuberculosis in humans. Where efforts have been made to identify the *Mycobacterium* species involved in human tuberculosis, *M. bovis* has been detected as a cause of both pulmonary and extrapulmonary tuberculosis in some, but not all, settings. One study has reported the isolation of *M. bovis* and *M. africanum* from 13% of human tuberculosis cases in Nigeria (*173*). In rural United Republic of Tanzania, *M. bovis* was identified in 4% of the culture-positive pulmonary cases (*174*) and from 10% of extrapulmonary tuberculosis human cases (*175*). It is recognized that care needs to be taken in the assessment of country situations, as findings may differ significantly between regions and ethnic groups (*171*). For example, *M. bovis* was isolated from 6.9% of tuberculous patients in a pastoral community in Uganda (*176*), whereas a study in a different rural community failed to detect *M. bovis* from 70 culture-positive cases of pulmonary tuberculosis, despite a high frequency of raw milk consumption and high prevalence of infection in cattle in the region (*177*). In Taiwan, China, only 0.5% of isolates (15 out of 3321 isolates) were characterized as *M. bovis*, with almost all (14/15) derived from patients with pulmonary tuberculosis (*178*).

The disease burden of *M. bovis*, calculated as DALYs, has been estimated in United Republic of Tanzania as approximately 1.3% of the total burden of tuberculosis in the country (*179*). However, this estimate was based on limited data and substantial efforts are still needed to provide rigorous estimates of the burden of disease. Further research is also needed to understand the specific risk factors for zoonotic transmission, with only limited analysis of risk factors associated with *M. bovis* infection in humans carried out in United Republic of Tanzania (*175, 180*) and Taiwan, China (*178*). Many questions remain about the significance of other non-tuberculous *Mycobacterium* infections, which are frequently isolated from both pulmonary and extrapulmonary TB patients. For example, non-tuberculous *Mycobacterium* species were isolated from 50% of culture-positive cervical lymphadenitis cases in rural communities of both United Republic of Tanzania (*175*) and Uganda (*176*) and from 25% of mycobacterial lymphadenitis cases in children in India (*181*). Despite evidence that non-tuberculous *Mycobacterium* may be posing a substantial, and growing, threat to human health, virtually nothing is known about these infections in terms of burden of disease, transmission routes, risk factors and implications for treatment outcomes.

3.2.3.4 Anthrax

Anthrax is caused by *Bacillus anthracis* and is endemic in herbivorous animals in the tropics. The bacterium lives in soil and is ingested while animals are feeding or by exposure to heat-and desiccation-resistant spores, which can live for decades in the environment, by entry of spores through the skin, by inhalation or by consumption of contaminated meat. The treatment of patients is based on the use of high-dose antibiotics, i.e. penicillins or cotrimoxazole. Although anthrax has been ranked as a high-priority disease in terms of animal health and poverty (*182*), little information is available about the true scale of the human disease problem. Hospital data from Africa are largely restricted to information on cutaneous anthrax, presumably because acute infections causing pulmonary or gastrointestinal anthrax have high case-fatality rates and victims invariably die at home before being able to reach hospital. Research on human anthrax needs to address several major data gaps with studies generating information on: (1) the incidence of human disease and deaths (for cutaneous, pulmonary and gastrointestinal forms of the disease); (2) the DALY and economic burden; (3) risk factors for infection and different forms of the disease; (4) the development of appropriate methods for diagnosis and surveillance. Preliminary data from United Republic of Tanzania indicate high anthrax seroprevalence levels in domestic dogs in anthrax-affected areas, suggesting that dogs may have utility as proxy or sentinel populations for disease surveillance where disease reporting is lacking, and may be used to examine environmental risk factors for infection.

3.2.4 Viral infections

3.2.4.1 Rabies

Rabies is a viral disease that is almost always fatal within a few days once clinical signs occur. The virus belongs to the genus *Lyssavirus*. Although rabies circulates in a number of domestic and wild carnivore and bat species, infection cycles are maintained by distinct species in different geographical areas (e.g. dogs in much of Africa and Asia; raccoons in the eastern USA; foxes in eastern Europe; yellow mongooses in South Africa). Infection of humans follows bites by rabid animals. More than 90% of all human rabies cases result from contacts with dogs in the developing world. Suspicion of infection in humans and animals is based on symptoms and signs, supported by epizootiological information. A confirmed diagnosis is made using standard laboratory tests carried out on tissues, mostly of nervous system origin and usually collected post mortem. Rabies has a wide geographical distribution and is present on all continents except Antarctica. A number of countries (mainly islands and peninsulas, for example in the Caribbean, the Pacific Ocean and the Mediterranean) are, however, recognized as free of the disease. Canine rabies is present in most of Africa, Central and South America and Asia, where the highest burden of human rabies is found. Rabies in dogs poses a threat to more than 3.3 billion people. It is estimated that 55 000 people die from dog-mediated rabies annually in Africa and Asia (*13*).

Where rabies is a public health problem, prevention of the disease in humans depends on a combination of interventions, including control of rabies in the animal reservoir, primarily the domestic dog in countries where the vast majority of human deaths still occur. Additional measures include pre-exposure immunization of humans at occupational risk of contracting the disease and on the speedy delivery of post-exposure prophylaxis (PEP) to potentially exposed patients (*183*). Theoretical and empirical studies suggest that the immunization of 70% of the dog population is effective in preventing rabies outbreaks in populations at risk (*184–186*). The key to the success of vaccination programmes is knowledge of the ecology of the dog population and the nature of human/dog interactions in the area.

To date, only a few studies of human disease incidence are available for developing countries (*34, 187*), and widely cited figures for human rabies mortality and DALY burden in Africa and Asia have relied upon estimates generated from the incidence of animal-bite injuries and rates of post-exposure vaccination (*13*). These estimates suggest that 1.8 million DALYs are attributable to rabies, although, with the rapid growth of dog populations in Africa and Asia, and an increasing incidence of dog rabies in many countries, revised estimates are likely to indicate a major increase in the DALY burden.

Rabies is predominantly a disease of children, with children between 5 and 15 years at highest risk. This is because children are more often bitten than adults and, when bitten, are more likely to incur injuries in high-risk sites on the body, such as the head and neck.

National rabies control programmes based on mass immunization of dogs initiated in 1983 in Latin American countries have achieved considerable success, with human and dog rabies now eliminated from Argentina and Chile and from major urban centres of other Latin American countries. In 20 years of PAHO-coordinated activities, dog-transmitted human rabies cases have fallen by more than 90% (*188*), although high-risk foci still remain. For example, cases of rabies transmitted from vampire bats appear to be increasing in some areas, which has been attributed to environmental disturbance, migration and limited access to health care in remote regions.

4. Intervention-oriented research issues

4.1 Community-led or community-directed interventions

The Alma Ata Declaration in 1978, which promoted health for all and equity through the institutionalization of primary health care paved the way for people's participation in health care, planning and implementation. It called on all governments, international organizations and the global community to come together to provide the necessary health and social support to enable people to attain a level of health by the year 2000 that would allow them to lead a socially and economically productive life.

Although the Alma Ata Declaration was unable to meet its promise of attaining "health for all" by the beginning of the 21st century, it has spawned some models of community participation in making health products, technologies and services accessible, especially to the poorest populations in many developing countries. For example, the World Bank and WHO launched the African Programme for Onchocerciasis Control (APOC) in 1995 with the aim of establishing a sustainable community-directed delivery system of ivermectin to control human onchocerciasis (river blindness) in endemic African countries by providing millions of annual treatments. The programme utilizes the community-directed treatment approach, which is a sustainable and cost-effective mass drug administration for distributing donated ivermectin to treat onchocerciasis in areas of high and medium endemicity. This approach empowers families and communities, instead of the health services, to assume responsibility for obtaining and distributing drugs in their village/community settings. Local communities decide together how they will collect the tablets from the supply sources, when and how the drug will be distributed, who assumes responsibility for distribution and record-keeping, and how the whole process is monitored.

It is estimated that APOC saved 3 million DALYs between 1996 and 2005, and, with a free supply of ivermectin, this gives an estimated 17% economic rate of return on the cost of treatment delivery (*189*). The Programme has also yielded other indirect benefits, which include improved overall health in communities, deworming (an ancillary benefit of ivermectin), and improved school attendance and food production. APOC was found to be effective not only in controlling onchocerciasis but also in the implementation of other health programmes particularly for malaria, tuberculosis, vaccination and micronutrient deficiencies (*190*). A recent multicountry study demonstrates the value of the community-directed approach in delivering other health interventions, particularly in increasing bednet uptake and home-based management of malaria (*191*).

In terms of improved sanitation, a key factor for many zoonotic diseases, community participation, is essential to achieve sustainable change that will translate into better quality of life and better health status. In low- and middle-income countries, strategies to improve sanitation range from systematic approaches, such as the provision of potable water and installation of sewage systems and indoor plumbing, to more restricted interventions, such as the installation of community water wells and household latrines or toilets. The latter is a widespread intervention that has met varying degrees of success, as in many instances, the presence of latrines or toilets alone does not secure better family and/or environmental hygiene (*192*, *193*). Indeed, these studies showed that to have a positive impact in the prevention of diarrhoeal diseases in children, water supplies and sanitation needed to be accompanied by changes in domestic hygienic behaviour (*192*). Similarly, it was shown that there was a significant association between hygienic behaviour and the presence of adequate household excreta disposal facilities, thus demonstrating the synergistic effect of the two factors (*193*). More recently, however, a report from Brazil demonstrated that, socioeconomic factors, rather than the presence of water and sanitation, were associated with a large proportion of the diarrhoea burden in children under 10 years of age (*194*). These investigators pointed to the changing epidemiology of diarrhoea in the city of Salvador, where the expansion of the sanitation network and other efforts make it hard to pinpoint specific risk factors for diarrhoea such as deficient water and sanitation systems (*194*, *195*). A recent analysis of the literature shows that hand-washing with soap, improved water quality and improved excreta disposal reduce the diarrhoea risk by 48%, 17% and 36%, respectively (*196*). In view of this evidence, in resource-poor settings, where access to water is minimal, immediate efforts to reduce diarrhoea should focus on environmental sanitation and the elimination of open defecation. This can be achieved with full community participation through the utilization of various participatory methodologies. One strategy that focuses on this is known as Community-led Total Sanitation, which is discussed below.

4.1.1 Community-led Total Sanitation

Nearly 2.6 billion people have no access to adequate sanitation and instead are culturally habituated to defecate in the open. This massive faecal contamination of the environment leads to unsafe drinking-water and, compounded by a lack of access to health care, a serious risk to health. As a direct consequence, one child dies every 15 seconds from diarrhoeal disease transmitted through faecal contamination of the environment, water or food. Billions of dollars are being spent on construction of latrines, providing safe water and teaching hygiene to local communities. Unfortunately, these efforts often fail to produce any significant or sustainable improvement of sanitation or any reduction in diarrhoeal disease morbidity and mortality.

In recent years the development and scaling-up of a movement to create local community action to improve environmental sanitation has begun to reverse the situation. Termed "Community-led Total Sanitation" (CLTS), the approach was pioneered in Bangladesh and has subsequently been introduced in 34 other countries in Africa, Asia and Latin America. Already millions of people living in rural areas have been able to stop the practice of open defecation and improve other collective and personal hygiene behaviours. There are two different approaches, the "Target-driven Partial Sanitation" approach (which focuses on prescriptive technology, introduced from outside the community, including educational modules to improve hygienic behaviours) and the CLTS approach which focuses on local empowerment and capacity-building in order to motivate a community to achieve and sustain universal use of safe faecal disposal methods. Such communities are given "open defecation free" (ODF) status (*197*). The CLTS methodology facilitates the capacity of a community to analyse its sanitation profile and practices of defecation, and to consider the health consequences. It is oriented towards voluntary commitments to collective action to become ODF (*197*). Stopping open defecation is the starting point to sustainable hygiene and behaviour change, and can be followed up with measures to improve sanitation system hardware and the environment, while creating opportunities for livelihoods involved in sustaining these changes. CLTS never teaches, prescribes technologies or subsidizes sanitation hardware. It only engages local communities in collectively analysing their sanitation profile, identifying the problems and taking the necessary decisions to act.

4.1.2 CLTS and zoonotic diseases

Many of the zoonotic diseases are transmitted from vertebrate animals to humans, humans to humans, or even humans to animals via soil and water contaminated with faeces from infected individuals. Although there is no systematic research thus far to assess the impact of CLTS and ODF status of communities on the incidence and prevalence of these infections, there is every reason to believe that a cleaner environment will reduce transmission of these infections, as well as bacterial and viral diarrhoeal infections, parasitic zoonoses and soil-transmitted helminths. Because of the persistence of infectious forms of some zoonotic infections and the soil-transmitted helminths, the most immediate effects are likely to be on the frequency of diarrhoeal disease. Initial assessments of community acceptance have been conducted by the Institute for Development Studies at the University of Sussex (Chambers R. *Going to scale with community-led total sanitation: reflections on experience, issues and ways forward* (IDS Practice Paper 1)[1].

---

[1] http://www.communityledtotalsanitation.org/sites/communityledtotalsanitation.org/files/Chambers_Going%20to%20Scale%20with%20CLTS.pdf

This summarizes the methods and challenges of implementing CLTS in six countries. The present strategies of tackling zoonotic diseases focus on either treating infected humans or targeting animals by segregating/treating/vaccinating them. These approaches are often disease-specific, and reductions in prevalence or incidence are costly and logistically difficult to sustain. Fresh faecal contamination and continued transmission always takes place unless the basic hygiene behaviour is changed. Although the polio vaccine eradication programme, which relies entirely on vaccine delivery, has been highly successful, the results could have been enhanced by triggering CLTS in communities and encouraging them to become ODF to reduce the continued introduction of wild polio virus into the environment. Similarly, a transmission dynamics model of cysticercosis suggested that improved sanitation and restricting access of pigs to human faeces would be a more sustainable approach than pig vaccination and treatment combined with human treatment (*56*).

It remains to be evaluated whether the reduction in worm loads of helminthic infections associated with oral-faecal transmission can be achieved through cessation of open defecation and also have a definitive impact on the transmission of diarrhoeal disease agents. These potential impacts are summarized in Figures 5 and 6. Such evaluations should include villages that have achieved ODF status and those that are still moving towards 100% ODF. Full community sanitation of human faeces may not eliminate all infections, as animals closely associated with households may continue to be the source of human infection. However, the change in behaviour in ODF villages may energize other hygienic practices, including hand-washing and protection of household drinking-water and cooking water from contamination. Moreover, even during the time before conclusive evidence is obtained about the health impact of sanitation (*196*), activities to expand the CLTS approach should be continued. It is clear that environmental interventions can have a substantial effect on diarrhoea morbidity and mortality as well as other important benefits, including the enhancement of human dignity (*196*, *198*).

For rural communities that use human excreta as manure for agriculture, it is important to include an assessment of the dangers such practices represent, and at what stages of Eco-San (Ecological Sanitation) the manure could efficiently and safely be used.

CLTS has already had a profound effect on many communities in over 30 countries across three continents, enabling many millions of people in local communities to construct affordable toilets (Figure 6). In particular, it has reached the poorest families and communities, many of whom depend on livestock for their livelihoods and have little or no access to safe water or basic sanitation and health services. It fosters privacy and convenience especially for

Figure 5
Some of the major economic, health and social impacts of Community-led Total Sanitation

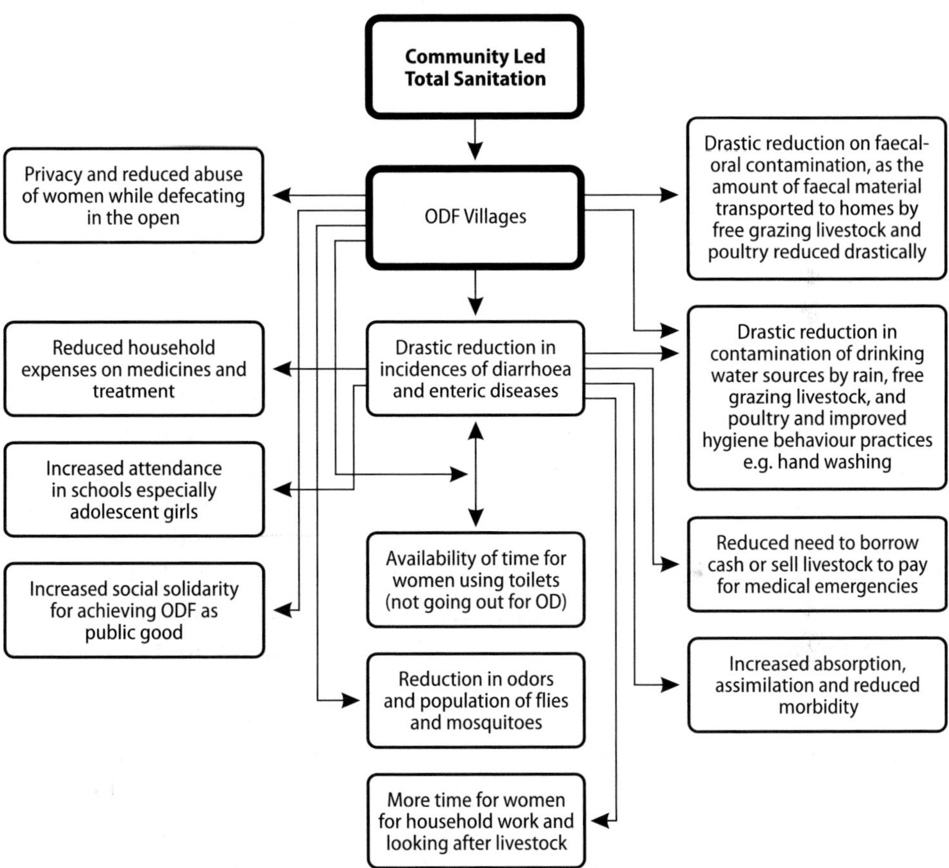

menstruating and pregnant women and among those in purdah. Furthermore, it can be quickly mainstreamed or scaled up by the government health systems in countries. Often the communities that achieve ODF status continue to develop other initiatives, as natural leaders emerge to solve other problems of rural communities. A similar experience has been seen in the onchocerciasis programme in Africa where additional health interventions are added to the ivermectin distribution package (*190*). Such approaches could include achieving "hunger-free status", thereby enhancing food security by eliminating seasonal hunger from the entire community, and ensuring improved school attendance with ensuing educational benefits, particularly for females.

Figure 6
Potential positive impacts of Community-led Total Sanitation on human health and possible impacts on diseases of the poor including zoonoses

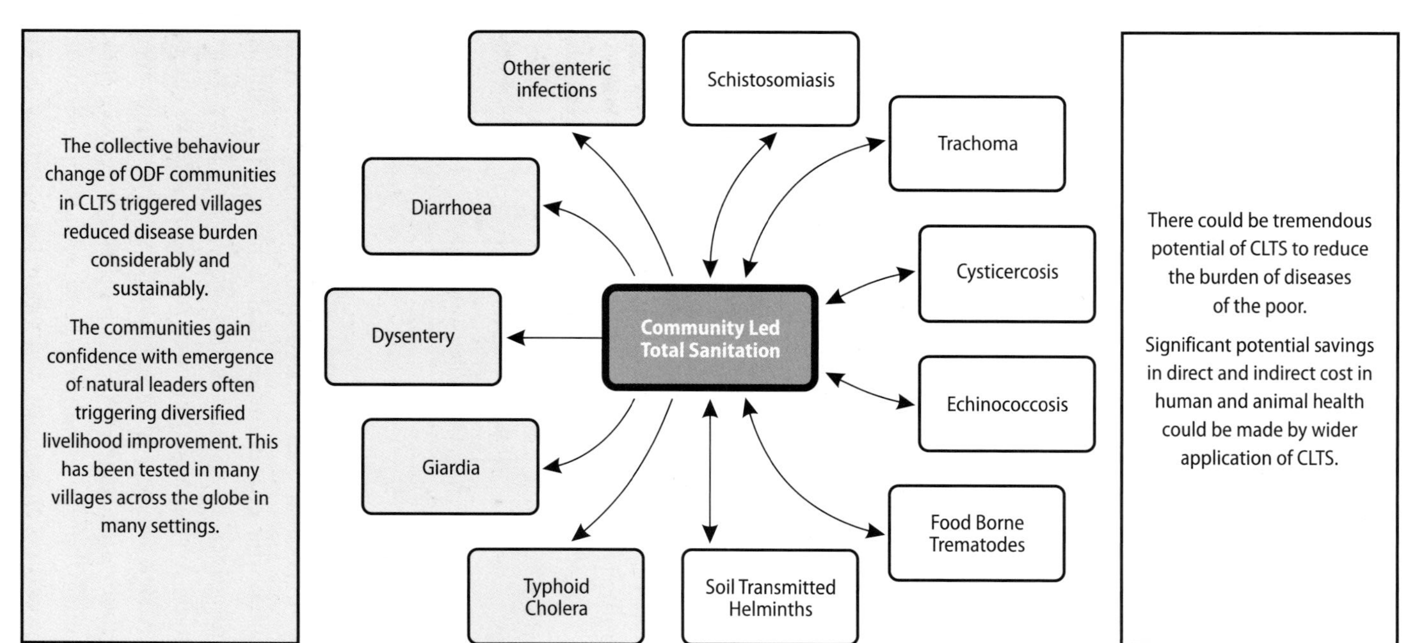

Previous vertical programmes to address diarrhoeal diseases have given way to the Integrated Management of Childhood Illness (IMCI). This includes broad messages on basic nutrition and micronutrient intervention programmes, administration of the routine vaccines included in the Expanded Programme on Immunization, and case management for acute respiratory and diarrhoeal diseases and malaria. Community-level water and sanitation interventions, as well as the necessary research investments in technology, community engagement, and behavioural change, remain relatively neglected and significantly associated with poverty.

Table 5 emphasizes the similarities and differences between three community-led or community-directed initiatives, which can be used to develop implementation research models of direct value to communities afflicted by zoonotic infections.

4.2 The human/animal interface: "One Health" as a concept

While recognizing that existing approaches to the control of and research into zoonotic diseases will continue to benefit from their current vertical or horizontal structure, there is growing evidence for the benefits of a joint human and animal health approach. The "One Health" concept, which involves a greater degree of integration of human and animal health resources, should be promoted, because many zoonoses can be better surveyed, diagnosed and controlled by considering human and animal health together. Such an approach would greatly facilitate detecting and addressing zoonoses. It would also ensure better access to health inputs for poor people and recognize the needs of their livestock. Encouraging cost-sharing in proportion to the benefits gained by each sector could be an enabling component of a "One Health" approach.

There is a need to generate data on the societal and economic impact of zoonotic diseases. This will require addressing the quantification of human morbidity and mortality (DALYs), impacts on livestock production, consequences for livestock trade (condemnation of carcasses), impacts on wildlife production and biodiversity, and social impacts (e.g. social stigma, fear) in a comprehensive way using examples such as cysticercosis, echinococcosis, brucellosis and rabies.

An additional component of animal diseases is the requirement to identify and quantify the component of the burden of disease due to the potential contribution of zoonotic diseases to non-communicable disease burdens. This is related in particular to neurological disorders, liver disease, cancer and injuries using case-studies of cysticercosis (epilepsy and headaches), echinococcosis and schistosomiasis (liver disease), foodborne trematodes (biliary and hepatic cancer), toxoplasmosis (schizophrenia, congenital/fetal abnormalities) and rabies (injuries).

Table 5
Comparative analysis of operational community-based interventions on health

Criteria	Community-led Total Sanitation (CLTS)	Community-directed Intervention (CDI) (ivermectin/albendazole)	Community-based Initiatives (CBI)
	Year of innovation	Year of innovation	Year of innovation
	1999-2000	1995	1988
Global spread so far	34 countries across south and south-east Asia, Eastern Mediterranean countries, eastern, southern, central and western Africa and Latin America	25 African countries	17 countries in Eastern Mediterranean Region (EMRO)
Adopted in the National Sanitation strategy of the governments of countries	at least five countries have adopted CLTS approach in their national sanitation strategy (Indonesia, Ethiopia, Sierra Leone, Zambia, Eritrea)	approach adopted as implementation platform in endemic areas of onchocerciasis and lymphatic filariasis	in the areas implementing the initiatives in EMRO region
Rough estimate of number of people benefitted	difficult to access but at least more than 10 million	75 million for onchocerciasis in Africa, and 80 million for lymphatic filariasis in Africa	18 million (about 5% of the total population of the region)
Perceived benefits	sharp decline in household medical expenses mainly through reduction in the incidences of diarrhoea, dysentery, cholera and typhoid	improved well-being, both physical and mental, and improved nutritional status	improved essential health indicators
Disease-specific benefits	sharp reduction in the incidences of diarrhoea, dysentery, cholera and typhoid	reduced blindness, skin disease, intestinal worm load, anaemia and frequency of filarial fever	decreased infant and child mortality

continues

Table 5 *continued*

Criteria	**Community-led Total Sanitation (CLTS)**	**Community-directed Intervention (CDI) (ivermectin/albendazole)**	**Community-based Initiatives (CBI)**
Rural communities access to interventions depends on:	their collective desire for hygiene behaviour change, starting with stopping open defecation	demand for donated efficacious products driven by community ownership	ownership of the community of the interventions
Outsider's role /Donor/ NGDO	facilitators of a process of empowerment and change	donor support for APOC; facilitators for creating awareness and process of empowerment	facilitators for creating awareness and process of empowerment
Insider's role	active analysis of their own sanitation situation, planner and implementer of CLTS to achieving ODF status as soon as possible	realization of the need for community distributor as leader of the process	taking active role in managing integrated development
Expected early outcome	"open defecation free" communities	community-managed drug distribution system working	functional community leadership
Time needed to get the first outcome	anything between 1 and 2 weeks to 3 months depending on the size of community and other factors	rapid impact of drug on skin itching and de-worming	about a year
Inputs supplied by outsiders	hands-off facilitation only	donated drugs, Training by NGDOs partners	training and interest-free loan
Prescriptions of technology or practice	nil at the outset; only on demand later	training, evaluation and reporting of coverage	CBI guidelines

continues

Table 5 *continued*

Criteria	Community-led Total Sanitation (CLTS)	Community-directed Intervention (CDI) (ivermectin/albendazole)	Community-based Initiatives (CBI)
Sustainability depends largely on:	insiders; their collective desire for maintaining ODF status	perceived value of drugs	on the community
Spread and scaling up by:	self-spread to neighbouring communities; natural Leaders emerging from ODF villages, NGOs, government field extension staff	advocacy at all levels; national and NGDO commitment	self-spread to neighbouring villages and NGO staff
Informal indicators of change from community perceptions	reduction in the population of flies and mosquitoes, sharp fall in the number of diarrhoea patients visiting village doctors and health centres, rise in the sale of sanitation hardware in village and nearby markets,	demand for continued annual drug distribution; continued high coverage at epidemiological level necessary	
Social solidarity	better-off members of the community contribute voluntarily to the poor to achieve ODF status, which is a 'public good' and not a 'private good'	CDD selected by community as leaders;	very high
Cost of implementation	low to very low	costs borne by community; principle of no remuneration	relatively low

continues

Table 5 *continued*

Criteria	**Community-led Total Sanitation (CLTS)**	**Community-directed Intervention (CDI) (ivermectin/albendazole)**	**Community-based Initiatives (CBI)**
Time taken to initiate the process	3 to 4 hours trigger CLTS in communities and follow-up until ODF status is reached	1-2 days training	1-3 months
Chances of continuing with other community led initiatives	fairly high as the local communities initiate actions in other areas of sanitation or livelihood development	extensive opportunity for CDDs to participate in other health interventions; upscaling of bednet uptake; home-based malaria management	
Sustainability index	fairly high to medium	high to medium; accessed through standardized process	high
Informal indicators of change from community's perceptions	reduction in the population of flies and mosquitoes, sharp fall in the number of diarrhoea patients attending health facilities	maintenance of commitment to collect drugs	

4.3 Chemotherapy and immunization

4.3.1 Mass chemotherapy (mass-targeted, humans-animals)

In the context of the parasitic and bacterial diseases, chemotherapy plays a significant role in curative approaches to individual therapy and in some situations in mass drug administration (MDA; preventive chemotherapy). Whilst these are well known and there are tested drugs to combat trematode and cestode infections (praziquantel in particular), there are also definitive needs for improved drugs or drug combinations, regimens and dosages to improve efficacy or reduce the risks of transmission. For the treatment of non-zoonotic neglected diseases, the majority of which are based on donation programmes, WHO has developed a handbook on preventive chemotherapy (*199*) recommending the strategies required in different endemic areas where several infections may be co-endemic and where the treatment frequency may vary from annual to semi-annual. However, this approach has not been applied widely to control zoonotic helminth infections, although mass distribution of praziquantel has been used in China and the Philippines for the control of *Schistosoma japonicum* and successfully for the elimination of *S. mekongi* in Cambodia (*80*). It is also applicable for the control of the foodborne trematodes (*200*), specifically for clonorchiasis, opisthorchiasis and *Paragonimus* at a single oral dose of 40 mg/kg. These diseases are being targeted in Lao People's Democratic Republic and Viet Nam following pilot studies in 2007 (*201*). The challenge is the high cost of praziquantel, although in recent years the cost has been driven down considerably and the unit cost per individual treatment is now around US$ 0.32 (*3, 202*). An example of the use of the principle of MDA for a zoonotic disease using a donated product is the distribution of triclabendazole (donated by Novartis). This drug is used as a curative treatment and is registered in only four countries: Ecuador, Egypt, France and Venezuela. The recommended single dose of 10 mg/kg makes this drug useful for the MDA approach, and mass drug distribution of triclabendazole is currently ongoing in areas of endemic fascioliasis in Bolivia and Peru. The WHO website www.who.int/neglectedtropicaldiseases provides information on fascioliasis and how countries may apply for donations of triclabendazole. The WHO policy on the control foodborne trematodes is summarized in reference 201.

For the treatment of the cystic stages of echinococcosis in humans, there has been limited progress in improving on the current regimes of long-term relatively high-dose treatment with albendazole (10 mg/kg per day) or mebendazole (40 mg/kg per day). These drugs severely damage cysts but are parasitostatic rather than parasiticidal. Albendazole is the more efficacious due to its better absorption. A third of cystic echinococcosis patients have been cured through chemotherapy using benzimidazole drugs and many have seen cysts reduced in size (*203*). Long-term use of these drugs also inhibits larval development of *E. multilocularis* and reduces metastasis, thereby enhancing the survival of patients.

For infections of dogs with adult tapeworms, mass treatment with praziquantel (5 mg/kg) remains the treatment of choice (*204*) in combination with other approaches as applied in successful control campaigns in Cyprus, Iceland and New Zealand. Hydatid disease represents an excellent example of successful integrated control to reduce a public health risk. Deworming of the dog population contributes significantly to that end, especially when linked to health education, control of offal disposal, carcass condemnation, and other appropriate slaughter practices.

Chemotherapy has been used in a pilot trial in 12 villages in Peru for the control of cysticercosis using two rounds of oxfendazole (30 mg/kg) in the treatment of pigs to kill cysts and praziquantel (5 mg/kg) to target the adult tapeworms in humans. Previous trials with oxfendazole at lower doses were less effective in killing cysts and treatment coverage of the human population with praziquantel was around 75% (*54*). There was a reduction in both prevalence and incidence after the treatment, but the parasite was not eliminated and instead it stabilized at slightly decreased rates. However, a recent study in Cameroon using the TSOL18 vaccine in pigs and the treatment of pigs with oxfendazole demonstrated the potential for eliminating the infection by combined approaches (*205*). The study in Cameroon did not treat humans with praziquantel for the adult *T. solium* but interventions targeted to both pigs and humans should certainly have an enhanced impact on transmission parameters.

4.3.2 Immunization against rabies

Rabies differs from most other infections in that clinical disease can be prevented through timely immunization, even after exposure to the infecting agent. Rabies post-exposure prophylaxis (PEP) consists of local treatment of the wound, which should be initiated as soon as possible after a bite, followed by the administration of passive immunization with rabies immune globulin, if indicated, and a potent and effective rabies vaccine for active immunization. Widespread immunization of humans following exposure has significantly reduced the number of human deaths from rabies. More than 10 million people receive such prophylaxis annually, the majority living in China and India. In Africa and Asia, the number of PEP regimens delivered is estimated to prevent approximately 330 000 deaths (*13*).

PEP accounts for 80% of the estimated annual cost (US$ 600 million) of rabies in Africa and Asia. In the most rabies-affected areas, patient-borne costs for PEP account for nearly half the total costs of rabies treatment. The frequency of PEP is expected to rise dramatically in all countries with dog rabies, particularly in countries that are replacing vaccines derived from nervous tissue with the safer and highly potent cell-culture vaccines (*13, 33*). Preventive immunization is recommended for anyone at continuous, frequent or increased risk of exposure to rabies virus, by nature of either their residence or their occupation (e.g. laboratory workers dealing with RABV and related lyssaviruses, veterinarians, and animal handlers). Travellers with extensive outdoor exposure in rural high-risk areas, where immediate access to appropriate medical care may be limited, should also be vaccinated pre-exposure. Children living in or visiting rabies-affected areas are at particular risk.

4.4 Vector and intermediate host control

Vector control has played and continues to play a major role in the control of both endemic diseases (for example, malaria through long-lasting impregnated nets and indoor residual spraying) and epidemic diseases (e.g. dengue) of poverty which are transmitted by insects as well as other arthropods (e.g. ticks for relapsing fever). Snails may be considered the "vectors" for the transmission of all trematodes. They play the role of obligatory intermediate hosts where complex life-cycles result in the production of human and animal infective stages.

Historically, there has been recognition that snail control can contribute to the reduction in exposure and transmission of snail-borne diseases, specifically schistosomiasis, through chemical use as well as environmental modification (*207*). The widespread use of molluscicides has, however, lost favour because of environmental concerns and the costs and sustainability of the approach as mass or targeted chemotherapy of the human definitive hosts for schistosomiasis has been introduced. However, focal mollusciciding may still play role in particular epidemiological settings, such as the marshlands of southern China where geospatial methodologies can be used to predict the location of snail habitats and hotspots of transmission. In Africa where there is limited zoonotic-associated transmission of schistosomiasis (*S. mansoni*) there have been large-scale attempts to control the disease through integrated snail control by environmental management and the use of molluscides, although permanent reductions in transmission have not been achieved (*202*).

The Blue Nile Health Project (BNP) in Sudan was initiated in 1979 to develop better strategies for controlling the major water-associated diseases in tropical irrigation schemes. It has been estimated that the 10-year programme cost some US$ 154 million (1978 prices). The Gezira, Managil and Rahad irrigation systems were selected to represent typical irrigation systems throughout Africa and the Middle East, where malaria, diarrhoeal diseases and schistosomiasis are endemic, and as the areas most urgently in need of disease control in Sudan. In 1986, a study undertaken by the BNP on snail control was applied as part of a local *S. mansoni* control programme in a primary health-care setting in the Dalati and Agallu Metti areas of the Ethiopian Blue Nile Valley. Niclosamide was applied focally wherever infected snails were found and the monthly snail surveillance continued until 1989. As a result, overall snail infection prevalences were reduced from 11.2% (Dalati) and 32.0% (Agallu Metti) to zero and 2.0%, respectively. In 1989, the human prevalence of schistosomiasis was only 8.6% in Agallu Metti. This programme demonstrated that while it is feasible to control *S. mansoni* by implementing snail control strategies through the primary health-care system (*208*), maintaining the success achieved by large-scale yet pilot projects and the extension and funding support required for national programmes have not been forthcoming.

There have been no attempts to initiate snail control for the intermediate hosts of foodborne trematodes (*95*). The methods used for control of the water-associated diseases emphasize that permanent improvements in water supply and sanitation, in environmental and agricultural practices, in health education and community participation, and in primary health services can lead to a reduction in dependence on pesticides and drugs while achieving effective control.

4.5 Vaccination as a control option for zoonotic diseases

Globally, vaccines are considered the "magic bullet" for public health interventions in the control of infectious diseases, and this has been substantiated by the results of the WHO Expanded Programme on Immunization.

4.5.1 Animal-targeted immunization

Injectable vaccines for mass immunization of dogs against rabies were used for the first time in 1921 in Japan (*209*). Japan still enjoys the rabies-free status it acquired definitively in 1957. Malaysia initiated a rabies control programme in 1952 with compulsory vaccination of all dogs and rigorous destruction of ownerless dogs, which brought rabies under control within a year. During the second half of the 20th century, only a limited number of countries eliminated the disease in their dog reservoir using immunization as a main tool. These countries, in addition to those mentioned above, include Canada and the USA (in the 1950s), Taiwan, China, and Portugal (1961), Chile (1976) and Uruguay (1983). In 2009, the Pan American Health Organization/WHO Regional Office for the Americas initiated a programme for dog rabies control based mainly on mass immunization of dogs. Mexico, for example, vaccinated more than 10 million dogs a year. Dog rabies has now been eliminated from all major urban centres in other Latin American countries and accordingly human rabies has been reduced by more than 90%.

In China the annual number of human rabies deaths was reduced from 3300 in 2007 to about 2400 in 2008. This achievement mainly followed sustained campaigns for dog immunization and dog population control activities in the main infected provinces.

Parenteral vaccination of dogs against rabies is considered the most effective measure for controlling canine rabies. At least 70% of the dog population should be vaccinated in areas where canine rabies is endemic. High vaccination coverage can be achieved through swift campaigns involving intersectoral cooperation, community participation, involvement of local authorities in planning and execution, and media support. By the end of 2009, many developing countries in Africa (e.g. Angola, Morocco, South Africa, Tunisia, and United Republic of Tanzania) and in Asia (e.g. Indonesia, Philippines, Thailand and Viet Nam) had stepped up their dog rabies immunization programmes through vaccination to control dog rabies and thus eliminate human rabies.

North America and Europe independently proposed that mass immunization of the principal wildlife hosts against rabies might be more effective than culling. Oral vaccines were included in baits targeting the principal host species. In the early 1960s foxes in the USA were successfully immunized orally with live attenuated ERA virus. Other oral rabies vaccines were later developed, as well as systems for their mass production. The first field experiment was conducted in Switzerland in 1978 (*210*); this was followed a few years later by Germany and Italy, and by other European countries after 1985. Many western and central European countries that were previously rabies-endemic had been freed of rabies by 2008 as a result of successful oral vaccination programmes, e.g. Belgium, Czech Republic, Finland, France, Germany, Luxembourg, the Netherlands and Switzerland. When applied using the safest vaccine baits, oral vaccination of dogs (OVD) may increase dog vaccination coverage, particularly when applied in combination with parenteral vaccination[1]. However, OVD has not yet become an operationalized component of any dog rabies control and elimination programmes because of concerns over safety for humans and cost per vaccine bait.

Since *Schistosoma japonicum* is a zoonotic organism, a transmission-blocking vaccine for livestock could be implemented in countries where livestock animals play a major role in human infection (*211*). Indeed, randomized, double-blind trials in water buffalo, using DNA vaccines encoding *S. japonicum* antigens, have taken place in China, resulting in approximately 50% protection (*212*). As this exceeds the hypothetical level predicted by mathematical modelling (*213*) to reduce transmission significantly, a transmission-blocking vaccine could well be available and on the market within the next few years.

The recent landmark publication of the *S. mansoni* and *S. japonicum* genomes (*214*, *215*) takes us a step closer to the identification of further key protective epitopes and the development and implementation of effective anti-schistosome (non-zoonotic) vaccines. However, many research questions need

[1] http://whqlibdoc.who.int/hq/2010/WHO_HTM_NTD_NZD_2010.1_eng.pdf page 15

to be addressed if this goal is to be achieved (*86*). Vaccine development should be a priority along with other avenues of research in schistosomiasis, including the search for alternative drugs to praziquantel, as the future development of resistance against the drug cannot be ruled out.

4.5.2 *Echinococcus granulosus*

The successful CE control programmes show that prevention of transmission to either intermediate (ungulates) or definitive (dogs) hosts can reduce or even eliminate the infection in human and livestock populations. Hence, if one or both type of hosts could be vaccinated, an improvement in the effectiveness and speed of control would be expected. An *E. granulosus* vaccine would ideally prevent oncosphere development to hydatid cysts in sheep, and thus stop the development of adult gravid tapeworms in dogs. Mathematical models of CE control suggest that vaccination of sheep would be an effective control strategy, provided that over 90% vaccine coverage of the sheep population was achieved. This level of coverage is unlikely to be sustainable or realistic in developing countries. However, the most effective intervention revealed by the modelling was a combination of sheep vaccination and dog anthelminthic treatment. A vaccination coverage of about 75% in sheep and anthelminthic treatment of dogs every 6 months would still achieve a high level of control of disease transmission, thereby greatly reducing the cost of a control programme and probably also increasing compliance from dog owners.

Humoral immunity plays a major role in the natural host-parasite relationship in echinococcosis. This antibody response was used to develop the highly immunogenic recombinant vaccine, designated EG95, against *E. granulosus* (*216*). The vaccine has been shown to confer a high degree of protection against challenge with different geographical isolates of *E. granulosus*. This would indicate that it could have wide applicability as an effective tool for use in hydatid control campaigns, with the potential to prevent hydatid disease directly through vaccination of humans. Research into vaccination against established hydatid cysts, both as a treatment option and for use in conjunction with oncosphere vaccines, is needed to reduce the time required to break the transmission cycle of the dog–sheep strain (*217*).

Although the EG95 vaccine against ovine hydatidosis is a reality that now requires innovative delivery strategies (*217*), no similarly effective vaccine exists against canine echinococcosis. This is not because of the lack of potential for application, because such a vaccine for dogs would be of enormous benefit in further reducing the effective period required to stop transmission of *E. granulosus*. Rather, the scarcity of vaccine candidates for immune protection against the adult tapeworm infection reflects the lack of research on specific immune correlates, the lack of evidence until recently of natural immunity in dogs, and the difficulties and cost of maintaining experimental canids (*217*). Experiments to induce immunity in dogs through vaccination have been carried out (*218*, *219*) but have been questioned methodologically (*220*). Clearly, these experiments need to be repeated, confirmed and extended, and this research area warrants strong encouragement for the future.

4.5.3 Vaccine against *Taenia solium*

A prophylactic recombinant protein vaccine (TSOL18) against *Taenia solium* has been developed for use in pigs. A pilot field trial of the TSOL18 vaccine was recently undertaken in Cameroon (*205*). Two hundred and forty piglets 2–3 months old were distributed to 114 individual households in pairs. Vaccinated animals received three immunizations with 200 µg TSOL18 plus 5 mg Quil A and 30 mg/kg oxfendazole at the time of the second immunization. Necropsies were undertaken when the pigs were approximately 12 months of age. Viable *T. solium* cysticerci were identified in 20 control pigs (prevalence 19.6%) whereas no cysticerci were found in any of the vaccinated animals ($P<0.0001$). Combined application of TSOL18 vaccination and a single oxfendazole treatment in pigs has the potential to control *T. solium* transmission in endemic areas and, indirectly, to reduce the number of new cases of NCC in humans. An authoritative assessment of all the options for control and possible eradication using the different strategies has been provided in a summary study (*221*). However the cost–effectiveness, cost–benefit and sustainability of such an approach for developing countries still need to be determined.

4.5.4 Foodborne trematode vaccines

Recent reports indicate that fascioliasis is becoming a serious public health problem, especially in South America, Egypt and the Islamic Republic of Iran (sporadic cases are also on the increase throughout Europe). Vaccines targeted at animals could play an important role in controlling fascioliasis in animals and, by blocking transmission of infection, have a beneficial effect on disease in humans. A number of prototype anti-*Fasciola* vaccines are being developed (*222*, *223*) but no commercial product is yet available. There has been very limited interest in developing vaccines against other foodborne trematode diseases, such as clonorchiasis and opisthorchiasis.

4.6 Human-targeted vaccines

4.6.1 Enteric infections

Progress in the development of operationally useful vaccines for the range of enteric infections has been steady. However, with two notable exceptions, no new vaccines are ready for introduction as public health tools. One exception is rotavirus vaccines, already marketed and used in developed countries; the second is heat-killed whole-bacteria oral cholera vaccines, currently used in limited settings. Recent trials of rotavirus vaccines (*224*) have documented a reduction in all-cause severe dehydration by 30% and for severe rotavirus gastroenteritis by 61% in Malawi and 77% in South Africa (pooled vaccine efficacy of 61%). Of the 4417 infants included in the efficacy analysis, severe rotavirus gastroenteritis occurred in 4.9% of the infants in the pooled placebo group and in 1.9% of those in the pooled vaccine group (vaccine efficacy, 61.2%; 95% CI: 44.0-73.2). Although vaccine efficacy was lower in Malawi than in South Africa (49.4% vs 76.9%), the number of averted episodes of severe rotavirus gastroenteritis was greater in Malawi than in South Africa (6.7 vs 4.2 cases per 100 infants vaccinated per year). The pooled efficacy against all-cause severe gastroenteritis was 30.2%. The reduced efficacy in developing versus developed countries needs to be better understood to optimize the impact of rotavirus vaccines. Surveillance studies in rural China have estimated the incidence rate of rotavirus diarrhoea to be 61.4 cases per 1000 children per year in those under 5 years old. Extrapolating to a cohort of 5000 Chinese newborns, universal rotavirus immunization would prevent 1764 cases of rotavirus diarrhoea, with 882 hospitalizations averted (*84*). At 2004 prices, net savings were calculated to be US$ 14 112 from a societal perspective and US$ 34 751 from a patient perspective.

With subsidies from GAVI vaccine purchase funds, the price of already marketed vaccines has been reduced to US$ 0.15–0.30 per dose (*225*). This is inexpensive enough to be used in developing countries until the promising and even less expensive rotavirus vaccines under development in China and India are thoroughly tested and marketed (*226*, *227*). Since there are reasons to believe rotavirus vaccines will be widely introduced into developing countries in the near future, this report does not discuss rotavirus in detail. However, it is an example of the potential of highly effective vaccines to reduce morbidity and mortality due to specific enteric pathogens.

Two oral cholera vaccines based on heat-killed vibrios, with or without recombinant cholera toxin B subunit included as an adjuvant, have been shown to be safe, effective in well-designed controlled field trials, and feasible for use in the community (*228*). One, consisting of a killed whole cell plus recombinant cholera toxin B-subunit (WC/rBS), has been prequalified by WHO, and is licensed and sold in over 60 countries as Dukoral, primarily for travellers to cholera-endemic countries. It is administered in two doses 10 days apart and elicits protective efficacy 10 days after the second dose; the cost is approximately US$ 40 per dose. Overall protective efficacy as high as 85–90% has been demonstrated, lasting for at least 6 months among all age groups, but declining rapidly thereafter in children below 5 years of age. The second vaccine is a similar product containing both O1 and O139 *V. cholerae* serotypes but no recombinant B subunit (*229*). It has been produced, licensed and used only in Viet Nam, but more recently it has been reformulated under GMP conditions by the International Vaccine Institute (*230*), and this version has been submitted to WHO for prequalification. It has been licensed in India by Shantha Biotech as Shanchol and is now marketed in India for around US$ 6 per dose. The vaccine has shown longer-term protection in children under 5 years, although it appears to be less protective than Dukoral (*231*). Wider use of these vaccines in endemic areas, as well as pre-emptive use when the risk of potential epidemic spread is high, has been recommended (*232*). In cholera-endemic countries, vaccination should be considered as an additional tool to control cholera and therefore targeted at high-risk populations.

Vaccine development for shigellosis has been disappointing, as the most effective vaccines are also the most reactogenic, and therefore no candidate *Shigella* vaccine has yet been seriously considered for scale-up and implementation. This is, in part, because there are multiple species and serotypes of *Shigella* able to cause human illness. In addition, although immunity is known to be serotype-specific, the nature of protective immunity required for an effective vaccine remains unclear (*233*). Many approaches have been investigated, including oral immunization with live attenuated *Shigella* or *S. typhi* expressing *Shigella* O-antigens (*234*), isolated *Shigella* cell-surface components (*235, 236*), or parenterally administered *O*-polysaccharide-protein conjugates (*237*). To provide comprehensive protection against most *Shigella* species, serotypes and subserotypes (16 in all), a limited pentavalent vaccine containing *S. dysenteriae* type 1, *S. sonnei*, and *S. flexneri* 2a, *S. flexneri* 3a and *S. flexneri* 6 has been proposed (*238*), as the last three contain cross-reactive serotype-specific antigens for the remaining 11 *S. flexneri* strains. While this approach would simplify the development of a broadly effective vaccine for shigellosis, targeting the most common and most virulent species, the development of such a vaccine remains a daunting task.

4.7 Animal reservoirs

Targeting animal reservoirs to control zoonotic diseases has been a means of reducing transmission of infections to humans. An example of this strategy is the use of chemotherapy to reduce the animal reservoir of human sleeping sickness caused by *Trypanosoma rhodesiense* in Uganda (*239*). Although culling of domestic dogs is often carried out by veterinary and public health authorities as a response to rabies outbreaks, there is no evidence that culling operations today have any significant effects on rabies control. In addition to numerous practical, financial, demographic and ethical concerns relating to indiscriminate dog culling, major questions remain about the theoretical premise on which culling is sometimes justified. While the assumption that disease transmission is dependent upon host density (i.e. that disease transmission rates increase with increasing host densities) is intuitively appealing, there is no evidence for density-dependent transmission of rabies in domestic dog populations (*186*). Similarly, culling of wildlife has never provided an effective long-term solution to wildlife rabies control. The high reproductive potential of reservoir populations, perturbation effects on movements and contact patterns, together with the capacity of the environment to provide food, water and shelter, most often render population control efforts futile. Empirical evidence from diverse settings across the world indicates that mass vaccination of reservoir hosts, whether domestic dog or wildlife populations, remains the single most effective approach to rabies control and elimination.

Other examples include the use of vaccines in dogs for rabies control, and the dispersion of baited oral vaccines for the fox population to control rabies in Europe. Following development of a vaccine for bovines for *Schistosoma japonicum* control, its use is under consideration in China and the Philippines but will depend on the proportion of human cases derived from the buffalo source. The effectiveness of any vaccine in such settings will depend on the proportion of infections in other reservoir hosts that cannot be vaccinated.

For echinococcosis and cysticercosis, targeting the major animal reservoirs, respectively sheep and pigs, has been investigated recently. In the former, the use of ovine vaccines has been tested and, in the latter, the use of oxfendazole to kill larval cysts, the source of human tapeworm infection. All these approaches, however, seem to require additional interventions to reinforce the impact of the primary intervention on the reservoir; hence the need for integrated approaches.

4.8 Health education and health literacy

Infectious diseases, particularly those in the category of neglected diseases, thrive in conditions of poverty and associated factors such as inadequate sanitation and lack of formal education (*3*). In turn, they perpetuate poverty, thus minimizing opportunities for development and education (*240*).

Education leads to multiple benefits, including access to better economic opportunities, and is strongly associated with better health outcomes such as decreasing rates of infant, child and maternal mortality (*241*). Education is thus an essential component for social change (*242*) and is a key strategy to end poverty and decrease the burden of disease. In the context of the Millennium Development Goals, "Education that reaches the poor can contribute to a more equal society" (*242*).

The World Health Organization has identified literacy as a key determinant for reducing health inequities in both rich and poor countries (*243*). Indeed, the number of years of schooling is positively associated with lower maternal mortality, and maternal education has a strong association with child health (*242*).

Studies on infectious diseases have shown that, among populations living in endemic communities, lack of education (as measured by years of schooling) and insufficient knowledge about the common diseases to which people are exposed are common risk factors for increased incidence and prevalence. For instance, in Honduras, *Taenia solium* infections have been found to be more prevalent among those with fewer years of schooling (*244*), while in rural Peru lack of education beyond elementary school was found to be associated with higher levels of human *T. solium* seropositivity (*245*). In China, a review of the socioeconomic determinants of *Schistosoma japonicum* found that in most reports a higher educational level was associated with lower exposure to infected water and therefore lower prevalence of infection (*246*). Equally, for enteric diseases, studies in Brazil provide further evidence that childhood diarrhoea is more likely in children whose mothers had a low level of schooling (*194*).

It is generally assumed that improvements in education and increased awareness through access to health information would lead to change in behaviour. However, any sustainable effect between educational strategies and changes in behaviour has been difficult to ascertain, particularly in short-term interventions. A study in Mexico showed that an educational intervention was successful in increasing knowledge of the transmission of *T. solium* (*247*). However, although some changes in behaviour were also observed, they were variable and not statistically significant at only six months post-intervention (*247*). A study on cystic echinococcosis showed that, although the vast majority of the study population recognized hydatid cysts, the mode of transmission and association with human disease was largely unknown (*248*).

Some studies show that the possession of appropriate background knowledge does not always predict better health outcomes or behaviour. This has been documented widely for chronic diseases (e.g. cigarette smoking and lung cancer) and sexually transmitted diseases, but only a few studies on the diseases within the scope of this report have documented a disconnect between knowledge and action. For example, a study on rabies in Sri Lanka demonstrated that, despite awareness and knowledge about the disease, there was no accompanying improvement in responsible behaviour with regard to dog ownership (*249*). This is also true for pig owners, who understand that their animals have more chances of acquiring cysticercosis by roaming free and scavenging for food. In trying to explain the discrepancy between knowledge and action in the latter example, it has been proposed that other factors such as economic incentives or health risk perceptions may play a prominent role (*250*). The protective effect brought about by knowledge and awareness may be minimized by environmental and infrastructural conditions and limitation of resources. In addition, individual decisions and actions may be not as effective if exposure is beyond the control of the individual. The power of education is conditioned by the political, social and economic circumstances in which people live (*242*).

In the example of porcine cysticercosis, the reasons why small-scale pig holders allow animals to roam free are seldom explored. Smallholders may lack land to set up a sty or resources to build it. An FAO report concludes that some livestock keepers are simply too poor and their operations too small to overcome economic and technical barriers (*251*). Moreover, too often smallholders struggle to feed their families and cannot afford to feed their livestock. Under these circumstances, keeping pigs in confinement is not a viable option. This could explain the observation in north-western Mozambique, where the prevalence of porcine cysticercosis among households with knowledge about the parasite was not different from those without such knowledge (*252*). Other zoonotic diseases can present an even more complex scenario where education and awareness play only a limited role. For instance, the control of *S. japonicum* in China is compounded by agricultural practices and the existence of an animal reservoir, namely water buffalo, which spend more time in the water than cattle and thus have more opportunities to contaminate the water. Therefore, in addition to health education and treatment for humans, strategies that include replacement or treatment of water buffalo and the use of a transmission-blocking vaccine will need to be implemented to maximize control efforts (*211*).

A further aspect that needs to be taken into consideration when analysing discrepancies between knowledge and action to reduce zoonotic disease burden is that there are several infections which for ethnic and cultural (including religious) reasons may play a more immediate role in transmission than schooling or awareness. Such is the case of certain foodborne parasites, for example, protozoa (e.g. *T. gondii*), trematodes (e.g. *F. hepatica*, *Opisthorchis*, *Clonorchis*, *Paragonimus*) and cestodes (e.g. *T. solium* and *T. saginata*) (*253*, *254*). Discrepancies between knowledge and action are documented in both developing and developed countries (*255*).

The variable results concerning the effectiveness of health education in communities endemic for the infectious diseases may also reflect the need for longer-term studies and optimized educational design as well as participatory research and innovative evaluation methodologies. For example, a 12-year pilot study for the control of *S. japonicum*, focused on health education and promotion (complemented with treatment of infected people with praziquantel), was able to achieve long-term positive changes towards control and adherence to treatment, particularly in women (*256*). With shorter-term studies, available evidence shows that when educational interventions are undertaken with full community participation, their results are more effective and may lead to lasting effects (*252*). In Nepal, making use of the first steps of the PRECEDE-PROCEED model (see below), the organizers were able to engage the community in identifying practices needing improvement to control porcine cysticercosis (*257*). Encouraging results have also been reported in the United Republic of Tanzania where the PRECEDE-PROCEED model was fully implemented (*258*). A health education intervention resulted in behavioural changes and decreased incidence of *T. solium* infections by nearly half 12 months post-intervention (*258*).

The PRECEDE-PROCEED model, widely used in health promotion, provides a comprehensive structure for assessing needs and implementing and evaluating interventions. It is based on the premise that health risks are caused by multiple factors, and so efforts seeking to effect change (behavioural, environmental, social) must be multidimensional, multisectoral and participatory (*259*). This model, however, is complex, requiring a high degree of professional involvement and an organized system. Outcome Mapping (*260*) can be used in a variety of situations to engage stakeholders (groups, communities or institutions) to define desired outcomes, implement strategies and measure progress. An advantage of Outcome Mapping is that, in contrast with the PRECEDE-PROCEED model that focuses on health outcomes, it allows assessing or measuring real-time progress, not just end-results. Instead of defining success as accomplishing the ultimate target goal (for instance the decrease in incidence of a disease; presence or absence of diarrhoea), the success of the programme can be monitored through the use of progress markers (e.g. changes in hygiene practices) and by recording a gradient of changes in behaviour towards the ultimate goal (*260*). Wider recognition is needed of the constructive effects of fostering empowerment and strengthening self-sufficiency among populations exposed to the zoonotic diseases.

Finally, recent work has shown that beyond *functional literacy* (i.e. the skills of reading and writing), *health literacy* is fundamental in empowering individuals and communities to take actions conducive to improving their own health and their social and physical environment (*261*, *262*). An increasing body of knowledge supports the role of health literacy in fostering positive health behaviours and practices for the prevention of chronic diseases (*262*, *263*) but little has been done to explore its role as an asset in ameliorating the burden imposed by infectious disease in the poorest of the poor. The problem is compounded when addressing zoonotic diseases, as the communities may be migratory, nomadic or isolated. They may have little access to formal educational structures and concepts, and may not be catered for by traditional government facilities.

4.9 Development of human resources

The implementation of effective, reproducible and sustainable health promotion strategies, including health education, requires strong leadership, continuing cooperation and a harmonized vision among different sectors in academia, government and civil society.

A recent report from the Institute of Medicine of the US National Academies of Sciences clearly identifies the global need for strengthening the professional workforce capable of conducting surveillance and initiating appropriate responses to infectious disease threats. Moreover, the report advocates training programmes that foster inter-disciplinarity as well as the participation of community and public health professionals (*166*). This training model is essential for a broader understanding of the causality of infectious disease and is the cornerstone of control and prevention strategies that target an integrated approach to health and should be at the core of professional and technical curricula (*264*).

In regard to the infectious diseases of poverty, health education and health literacy can play a fundamental role in the empowerment of disadvantaged communities in disease-endemic countries (*265*). By tailoring health messages to specific populations, educators, researchers and decision-makers are more likely to reach broader audiences and to effect change. For example, research focus groups studied a rural community in Honduras where porcine cysticercosis was prevalent and where pigs were roaming freely through the village. The study showed that the small pig-holders, who were mostly women, were not only not interested in pamphlets with health information, but also disliked pamphlets or handouts portraying them in cartoons, as they consider this a lack of respect.

These findings were considered in the design of a communication strategy that integrated the role of literacy, gender and daily activities, such as going to the market, into a health message to encourage a behaviour change. Thus, a family canvas shopping bag with a drawing of a piglet and the legend "a pig in a pen is a healthy pig" was distributed among women. The bag was received enthusiastically by the women and they used it proudly every day and explained its significance to others who were curious about it (Maritza Canales, unpublished data).

4.10 Integrated approaches

Disease control programmes are typically integrated as there is a need to link surveillance, monitoring and reporting all activities with actions taken by the health system. With zoonotic diseases and the diseases of marginalized populations, interventions typically are directed at both the human and the animal host. Such approaches may be biomedical (drug or vaccine), vector or intermediate host control (insects or snail), environmental, legislative (inspection and condemnation of infected products at slaughterhouses) or educational. Integration must also be across the human health and animal health sectors. The recent example of integrated control of schistosomiasis in China was referred to earlier. There are several other examples of integrated control of zoonotic diseases that demonstrate the importance of addressing both ends of the host spectrum, the vectors (if present), the environment and behaviour change.

Control measures already exist for several neglected zoonotic diseases such as rabies, anthrax, echinococcosis, cysticercosis and brucellosis. Interventions can be packaged through existing veterinary and public health structures. Several examples of major successful control programmes indicate that national, regional or even global control/elimination should be possible. This integrated approach can be extended to incorporate non-zoonotic public health problems prevalent in the same impoverished communities. However, the effectiveness of these interventions in reducing human infection for some of the diseases (e.g. cysticercosis, echinococcosis) remains unknown.

Depending on the characteristics of the human and zoonotic diseases prevailing in the area, control of the zoonotic diseases can be integrated and viewed within existing health and agricultural systems. "Control packages" for animal diseases, similar to school-based programmes for the control of certain human diseases in children, should be developed. These would reflect a change from single-disease/vertical approaches to more integrated health promotion by development of new packages addressing several disease/health problems. The development of such packages needs to be supported by operational research to assess their impact, safety and cost–effectiveness and by disease control and cost modelling exercises where appropriate.

These packages should target populations such as: 1) pastoral communities and remote sedentary rural populations in Africa and Asia; and 2) marginalized urban livestock producers. Together these represent a substantial proportion of the 600 million poor livestock keepers worldwide.

4.11 New products and strategies

There is universal recognition that more research should be conducted to improve and develop new disease control tools. However, diagnostic, curative, preventive and monitoring tools must be adapted to the conditions prevailing in developing countries and recognize the constraints of financing, affordability and delivery. There is unprecedented interest in research on diseases of the poor, although there is still only a disproportionately small amount for research on zoonoses. However, there is a degree of optimism that this research will yield products that can be developed rapidly, can be financed and deployed within health systems, and can yield beneficial widespread impacts on health. The needed research should be undertaken cooperatively at the international level, be multidisciplinary, involve both human and animal health research groups, and engage relevant stakeholders. It should focus on integrated interventions, rather than target a particular and unique biological target, since it is likely that the cost–effectiveness and cost–benefit of a broader approach will be more favourable. The concept of the "mono-intervention" approach is not likely to be productive in zoonotic diseases but this approach is usually the target-driven focus of research in biomedical areas.

For most diseases there is a need for development of affordable, rapid, reliable and robust diagnostic tools appropriate for both field and local health facility settings in almost all of the diseases considered by this report. These tools should also be considered in the context of surveillance and monitoring and evaluation tools. There is a need for development of innovative strategies for disease surveillance, including the use of sentinel populations (both human and animal), adopting new approaches in communication technology and analytical tools (e.g. text/data mining such as the USDA livestock disease alerts), participatory approaches such as the use of abattoir workers for surveillance, and mobile phone reporting (e.g. as used to report rabies exposures in Pakistan).

In any assessment of disease control there is always an interest in vaccine development. However, in the context of zoonoses the drive to develop new vaccines for interventions in animal populations, including multivalent vaccines, could be justified if combination vaccines given through the same delivery strategy were demonstrated to be effective. For example, combined rabies/echinococcosis vaccine for dogs and a combined echinococcosis/brucellosis vaccines for sheep would be attractive concepts for development.

From a strategic perspective, there is a need to develop community-led initiatives for surveillance, treatment, prevention and control of infectious diseases, recognizing the need for two existing major community-based initiatives to share experiences since control strategies for infections are often complementary. Specifically, the Community-led Total Sanitation project and the African Programme for Onchocerciasis Control (although onchocerciasis is not a zoonosis) should meet to explore lessons learned as well as the removal of obstacles to scaling up the two approaches through communities. A recent WHO/TDR multicountry study has provided strong evidence of the health delivery opportunities afforded (*266*).

Although both the biomedical and social sciences approaches to research are crucial, it is important to identify effective strategies for translating research findings into policy change and through this to generate sustainable financing for implementation at the necessary scale. This is a significant challenge under ordinary circumstances, but in times of global financial stress it becomes significantly more difficult. There is also a need for research into the sustainability of systems to identify strategies to maintain control and prevention beyond the term of donor support.

4.12 Health systems and interactions with other sectors: intersectoral dialogue

A significant part of the problem of neglected zoonotic diseases is the lack of communication and shared information among the relevant communities that need to connect with one another. The establishment of a scientific multidisciplinary intersectoral advisory committee to share and communicate information, especially within countries where the burden of those diseases is high, would be a major step forward. In addition, measures should be taken to raise awareness among policy-makers in all involved sectors and at all levels to inform decision-makers of the importance and impact of zoonoses and marginalized diseases. The responsible international agencies (WHO, FAO and OIE), as well as other stakeholders, need to take leadership in the sensitization of national governments and donor communities to the importance of zoonoses both as endemic impediments to development and as immediate threats to health. Given the limited resources typically available in poor countries, WHO, FAO and OIE need to determine how to help establish international resource centres to gather existing educational and advocacy material for zoonotic and marginalized diseases.

Beyond the information-sharing function, a system for recognizing and funding centres of excellence in zoonotic disease research that are linked to local public health systems would extend the capacity of local communities to address their own problems.

4.13 Cost–effectiveness analysis

Very few studies to evaluate the economic implications of alternative control strategies for zoonotic diseases have been performed. Such studies need to quantify the production losses, such as reduced fertility, milk or wool production, poor weight gain of food animals and organ damage, as they can impose significant financial losses on livestock keepers (*267*). This is essential if the true impact of these diseases is to be evaluated. Such losses are difficult to quantify in developing countries, in part because they are dependent on the type of production system in the community of interest. Often there are few formal markets and opportunities to replace animals, which further challenges the accurate assessment of lost revenue. Even where appropriate treatments are commercially available, poor-quality animal health services and low compliance will make it difficult to compensate for the cost of treatment by the subsequent return to health of the animal and its value to the farmer.

5. Disease-specific and intervention-specific priorities for research

5.1 Disease-specific research priorities

This report identifies applicable and relevant priorities for each zoonotic disease covered by the DRG, identifying the knowledge gaps in zoonotic disease research and presenting the priorities for research.

While many disease-specific and agent-specific research needs are detailed in the sections below, there are five common threads in the knowledge gaps that, if addressed, will help to target interventions and bring significant health improvement in a short time frame. These are:

- studies of disease burden in both humans and animals in both urban and rural settings in a manner that brings the human and veterinary health communities together;
- determination of the economic cost of these diseases for both the human and animal populations involved;
- studies of the efficacy of integrated interventions that address more than one disease and/or agent at the same time;
- determination of the cost-effectiveness of these interventions;
- studies on promotion of health literacy and social mobilization to ensure maximal engagement of the affected populations in the selected interventions.

5.1.1 Cysticercosis and taeniasis

The following research priorities were identified by the DRG:

- new drugs, rapid diagnostics, drug regimens and treatment follow-up for taeniasis and human cysticercosis;
- field-based randomized clinical trials to evaluate the efficacy of oxfendazole and its effectiveness with recombinant vaccines against porcine cysticercosis;
- detailed studies to elucidate the spectrum of symptoms, including stroke associated with NCC to inform burden of disease studies;
- development of immunological tests for diagnosis and biomarkers of infection status/exposure and for differentiation of *T. solium* and *T. saginata*;
- development and validation of transmission dynamics models to assess the cost–effectiveness and cost–benefits of alternative control strategies;

- development of audience-specific health education and behaviour change interventions; and assessment of their effectiveness together with gender-related correlates in intervention studies.

5.1.2 Echinococcosis

The following priorities were identified for echinococcosis research:

- measurement of the health and economic burden of echinococcosis caused by both *E. granulosus* and *E. multilocularis*, including productivity losses in humans and animals and cost–effectiveness of current control approaches;
- multicentric prospective evaluation of available clinical treatment options, including surgery, ultrasound, drug regimens (albendazole, flubendazole and ivermectin, including dosages and combinations);
- improved sensitive and specific diagnostics for early detection of *Echinococcus* infection including:
  - methods (imaging, serology) to assess parasite viability and/or progression of both cystic and alveolar disease;
  - comparison of the efficacy, sensitivity and specificity of copro-DNA tests to establish strain-specific detection for *E. granulosus* in dogs;
- further assessment of different vaccine strategies/options/combinations, e.g. a vaccine for ovine echinococcosis and development of a vaccine for use in definitive canine hosts;
- development and validation of better transmission dynamics models to assess the cost–effectiveness of alternative control strategies.

5.1.3 Asian schistosomiasis

The zoonotic schistosomiases, *Schistosoma japonicum* and *S. mekongi* in Asia could be locally eliminated because new tools (e.g. an effective vaccine for buffalo) are available. However, more studies are needed to determine the role of the variety of animals in transmission as reservoirs (buffalo or others such as dogs, cats or rats). This is especially the case in the Philippines, where the precise role of carabao (water buffalo) in the transmission of *S. japonicum* needs to be determined.

- Operational research is required on the cost–effectiveness of integrated control to establish optimum approach at scale in different geographical settings, including the value of transmission-blocking vaccines for use in buffalo or other mammalian hosts.

- Studies on the problems of coverage and compliance related to access to mass treatment in the Philippines (Samar province) in relation to animal reservoir diversity to define which zoonotic sources have an impact on the incidence of human infections.
- Studies on the impact of schistosomiasis on malnutrition and cognition are required in relation to single infections and polyparasitism.
- Improved diagnostic methods are required where schistosomiasis prevalence is low and as a surveillance tool in order to determine whether effective control has been achieved.
- Development of appropriate and gender-sensitive tools and methods is needed to assess the health and socioeconomic impact of control programmes on individuals and households.

5.1.4 Foodborne trematodiases

The DRG benefited from recent WHO and TDR meetings on this topic and review papers in constructing the following priority listing for foodborne trematodiases (*89*):

- estimation of the global burden of foodborne trematodiases;
- increased interest in the discovery and development of new diagnostic tools, vaccines and new trematocidal drugs;
- determination of how improved access to clean water, adequate sanitation and sewage treatment, and enhanced food safety measures have an impact on foodborne trematodiases;
- while chemotherapy-based morbidity control should serve as the backbone of control programmes in areas where foodborne trematodiases are highly endemic, integrated control approaches and intersectoral collaboration between public health and veterinary medicine warrant more attention, including considerations of feasibility, efficacy and cost–effectiveness;
- operations research on integrated control (mass treatment, education and behaviour change communication, community-directed/led strategies for health, sanitation and aquaculture management) in endemic communities and intersectoral collaboration between public health and veterinary medicine and public and private sectors in planning implementation, including food safety issues;
- analysis of gender (male and female) differentials on access to and compliance with FBT treatment;
- development of appropriate and gender-sensitive tools and methods to assess the socioeconomic impact of FBT on individuals, households, communities and societies;

- evaluation of national FBT disease surveillance, and its effectiveness in tracking FBT infections. Together with the surveillance of other zoonotic diseases, assess the impact of FBT and its control into the health education programmes for communities and schools, and its effect on the knowledge and practice of endemic communities to prevent and control FBT.

5.1.5 Toxoplasmosis

The following priority research needs for toxoplasmosis were identified:

- development of animal vaccines;
- development of new economic and safe diagnostic techniques for acute infection during pregnancy to detect toxoplasmosis in the mother and fetus;
- assessment of the cost–effectiveness of integration of existing serological test regimes into antenatal care programmes in low-income settings;
- development of cost-effective diagnostic and management protocols for CNS toxoplasmosis in high-risk HIV-seropositive patients;
- development of culturally acceptable health education programmes to improve food hygiene in the home, especially for pregnant women;
- quantification of the impact of improved water quality and sanitation on toxoplasmosis infection;
- quantification of the proportion of chronic abortions globally that are attributable to toxoplasmosis.

5.1.6 Cryptosporidiosis

The following research priorities were identified for cryptosporidiosis:

- document the burden of cryptosporidiosis in young children in developing countries;
- determine the extent of livestock as source of *Cryptosporidium* infections in humans in the developing world;
- enhance surveillance of infection prevalence in humans and livestock, and determine the short- and longer-term health and economic consequences for both populations;
- assess the impact of community-level water and sanitation improvements on the prevalence of human infection, in both urban and rural settings;
- identify agricultural practices that reduce the exposure of livestock to infection in order to interrupt transmission to humans;

- develop a livestock vaccine to block animal infection and consequently reduce the excretion of infectious cysts into the environment and transmission of infection to humans;
- continue to explore new drug candidates for use in the immunocompromised host.

5.1.7 Rabies

Human rabies incidence can be reduced by mass dog vaccination campaigns in combination with prompt and appropriate post-exposure prophylaxis (PEP) for people suffering animal bites and possible exposure to the rabies virus. Cross-sectoral evaluation of this approach has clearly demonstrated the cost–effectiveness of interventions in the domestic dog population (*268*). However, challenges remain in developing sustainable strategies to resource this approach, including cooperation between the health and veterinary sectors (*269*). Surveillance also remains a major constraint throughout much of Africa and parts of Asia. Relatively few cases of human and animal rabies are confirmed by laboratory diagnosis because of limited laboratory diagnostic capacity and the lack of submission of diagnostic samples from clinical cases (both humans and animals). In addition, clinical diagnosis can be problematic, particularly in malaria-endemic areas, where a proportion of childhood rabies deaths are misdiagnosed as cerebral malaria (*270*). The priorities identified by the DRG were both implementation policy and basic research, as these are interrelated.

The following actions are needed to reinforce the research agenda:

- strengthening of laboratory capacity for diagnosis and surveillance to generate accurate data on rabies incidence in order to guide control strategies and estimates of disease burden;
- prioritization and cooperation between health, veterinary and wildlife agencies;
- adoption of appropriate and effective methods for collection of samples for diagnosis of rabies in humans both post mortem (e.g. periorbital biopsies, (*270*)) and antemortem (e.g. nuchal skin biopsies (*271*)).

Specific research priorities identified were:

- more widespread use of existing techniques for field collection and storage of samples and tests for rabies diagnosis and surveillance (*269*), such as the direct rapid immunohistochemical test (*272–275*), and use of preservatives/specialized paper for stabilization of virus and RNA;

- development and evaluation of new technologies for integrated, real-time surveillance and response (e.g. mobile computing technologies);
- evaluation of the cost–effectiveness of different WHO-recommended pre and post-exposure regimens, including indirect costs associated with hospital visits;
- evaluation and implementation of new biological regimens for humans, including use of monoclonal antibodies as a cost-effective replacement for rabies immunoglobulin (*276*, *277*);
- establishment of reliable, economical and harmonized *in vitro* laboratory tests to ensure the quality and in particular the potency of rabies vaccines;
- development of innovative strategies for funding integrated and sustainable dog vaccination programmes, including education and social mobilization campaigns;
- development of combined approaches to dog rabies vaccination and immuno-contraception (*277*);
- investigation of the economics of dog oral vaccination strategies and identification of appropriate settings for implementing oral vaccination campaigns in dogs (*277*).

5.1.8 Bacterial zoonoses

Owing to limited clinical laboratory infrastructure, a definitive diagnosis for diseases such as bovine tuberculosis and brucellosis can rarely be confirmed in routine clinical practice. Existing serological tests for brucellosis carried out in hospital settings often perform poorly, with problems relating to both specificity and sensitivity (*278*). For anthrax, an additional cause of underreporting is the rapid onset and progression of pulmonary and gastrointestinal cases, which means that patients often die before reaching medical facilities.

The following research priorities for bacterial zoonoses were identified.

- Inexpensive, robust and reliable diagnostic tests are required for use in field and hospital settings. Where tests do currently exist, such as the single comparative intradermal test for bovine tuberculosis and serological tests for brucellosis, establishing locally appropriate cut-off points is important for acquisition of valid data to inform disease burden studies.
- There is a pressing need for cross-sectoral assessment of disease burden to allow for realistic evaluation of the cost–effectiveness of disease interventions.

- A common measure of zoonotic disease burden that incorporates human health indices, costs to the public health sector, monetary burden for the livestock sector and costs to the private sector needs to be developed.
- Ethnographic and participatory research approaches are needed to design relevant and understandable criteria for measuring impacts that incorporate a broader consideration of burden with consideration of the value of livestock for human well-being and development.

Several key questions need to be answered for zoonotic tuberculosis in Africa. The priorities are as follows:

- understanding of the human disease burden, and how and why the prevalence of human *M. bovis* and non-tuberculous mycobacterial infections varies in different communities;
- identification of animal-related risk factors for human infection with different mycobacterial species, including potential factors associated with small ruminants (*279*);
- clinical research on optimal drug treatment regimens for etiologically confirmed *M. bovis* and non-tuberculous mycobacterial infections;
- evaluation of the effectiveness of the standard DOTS regimen administered in cases of tuberculosis caused by *M. bovis* and non-tuberculous mycobacterial infections, as few cases are differentiated on the basis of culture results;
- development of effective livestock vaccines and vaccination strategies for *M. bovis*, as conventional test-and-slaughter approaches that have been used to control and eliminate infection in industrialized regions are unlikely to be feasible in most developing countries.

For both brucellosis and anthrax, livestock vaccines are available. However there is a need to ensure immunogenicity and vaccine quality, improve vaccine safety, and design and implement targeted vaccination strategies that will optimize the cost–effectiveness of interventions.

The following research priorities for brucellosis were identified:

- critically assess the immunogenic properties of currently available vaccines and their effectiveness in areas of high endemicity;
- improve the safety and immunogenicity of the current vaccines against *Brucella melitensis* and *Brucella abortus*;
- design diagnostic strategies to differentiate vaccinated animals from naturally infected animals in order to prevent unnecessary livestock slaughter;

- develop inexpensive and reliable diagnostic tests for use in local hospital and field settings;
- generate data and develop methodologies to allow an accurate estimation of the societal burden of brucellosis, focusing primarily on burden of disease in livestock and human populations;
- design and evaluate cost–effective livestock vaccination strategies and advocate "One Health" approaches to implementation at the policy-maker level (ministries of health and agriculture);
- develop approaches to raise awareness among physicians of the need for differential diagnosis of *Brucella* in cases of non-specific febrile illness.

Even without a specific detailed knowledge of risk factors, several health measures are likely to be effective in preventing transmission of bacterial zoonoses, such as boiling milk (to prevent brucellosis and *M. bovis* infection) and hygienic precautions when handling abortions and placental material (to prevent brucellosis and Q-fever) and the carcasses, skin and hides of livestock that have died (to prevent anthrax). Applied research is therefore needed on the development, implementation and evaluation of appropriate preventive health educational measures that are likely to provide a cost–effective means of reducing the burden of a wide range of bacterial zoonotic infections.

5.1.9 Enteric infections

Current gaps in knowledge represent barriers to improving the effectiveness of measures to interrupt the transmission of diarrhoeal and dysenteric diseases. These gaps span the range of "upstream technical" to "downstream applied" questions. The needs are:

- develop better methods for surveillance of human enteric infections, including syndromic classification and etiology if possible, based in representative community settings, both urban and rural, and across the whole age range;
- clarify the reservoirs for animal and human enteric infections and the pathways of transmission among animals, from animals to humans, from humans to humans and from humans to animals;
- after identifying critical points in transmission, develop interventions that will target the most effective transmission routes and markedly diminish, if not abolish, their efficiency;
- develop infrastructure and capacity to identify zoonotic enteric pathogens in the relevant animal populations;

- determine the economic burden resulting from infections in livestock, including illness and loss of markets and income from animals and the direct and indirect economic costs of foodborne illnesses;
- test simple cost-effective farming methods to prevent transmission of zoonotic infection to animals, crops and water supplies, and to humans, which will be applicable to small- and large-scale producers alike;
- develop ways to improve the communications between veterinary and human health professionals, to include integrated training modules and mechanisms for exchange of information;
- create joint veterinary/human health outbreak investigation teams, with access to quality laboratory capacity for diagnosis allied to enhancement of veterinary and human grassroots public health educational services (educational extension model) to improve animal and human health outcomes;
- implement ongoing surveillance for drug resistance and determine the most effective means to disseminate this information;
- develop strategies to control the delivery of drugs used for enteric infections without restricting access when these medications are urgently needed in order to increase appropriate use and delay the emergence and spread of drug resistance;
- identify the optimal investments in livestock animal and human primary health care capacity to ensure appropriate treatment as well as the use of effective prevention modalities;
- increase investments in new drug and diagnostic test research and development programmes;
- develop multivalent, low-cost, locally produced vaccines sufficiently effective to interrupt transmission cycles;
- create new approaches to community sanitation measures and the provision of clean water supplies.

5.2 Intervention-specific research priorities

5.2.1 Community-led Total Sanitation

The key research priorities emerging from the experience of CLTS to date are:

- measure the effectiveness of CLTS on incidence and prevalence of zoonotic and marginalized diseases through epidemiological studies and community-based randomized trials;

- estimate the duration of "open defecation free" (ODF) status following CLTS;
- estimate the cost–benefit of CLTS as compared with other approaches;
- study the human-animal interface to clarify the social, cultural, behavioural, economic and gender dimensions of improving community access to proper sanitation through CLTS;
- evaluate the impact of CLTS on specific communities dependent on equines and camelines, smallholder pig farmers and those dependent on aquaculture.

5.2.2 Animal/human interface

In the area of the animal-human interface the key research priorities identified are:

- further study mechanisms for coordinated public and animal health action within national government systems that comprise both the public health and animal health systems as a single entity on an equal partner basis;
- increase the level of priority accorded to zoonotic diseases by increasing advocacy and undertaking research to underpin the importance of zoonotic infections as drivers of poverty;
- extend the concept to cover diagnosis, data-sharing, monitoring and surveillance systems, training, interventions and delivery.

5.2.3 Epidemiological studies

Small-scale focused epidemiological studies should be undertaken to gather basic information for the design of control programmes and awareness generation and to support advocacy. Such studies should focus on the following:

- assessment of the DALY burden borne by individuals affected by the diseases;
- assessment of the monetary impact of the diseases to livestock and human productivity;
- study of risk factors in both people and animals with a view to successfully targeting at-risk groups for high-priority intervention;
- investigation of methods for quantifying the rate of underreporting of these diseases in humans;
- development of transmission dynamics models to predict the effectiveness of alternative control measures;

- cohort studies on several zoonoses in which the symptoms in humans appear several years after infection;
- randomized trials to estimate the effectiveness of alternative control strategies, including integrated/combined strategies.

5.2.4 Health education and promotion

The priority areas for research are the following:

- long-term (longitudinal) studies assessing health education "multi-packs", i.e. for diseases with similar or overlapping bio-social determinants;
- gender-sensitive approach to health education/promotion and behaviour change, e.g. the role of women, as they more often tend to be small livestock keepers;
- comparative studies on traditional versus participatory research;
- evaluation research (assessment of methodologies for programme/project evaluation);
- assess the specific contribution of educational components within integrated interventions.

6. Cross-Group issues and priorities

6.1 Interactions with Disease and Thematic Reference Groups

Involvement in the meetings of Chairs and co-Chairs, attendance at the Stewardship Advisory Committee and interactions with the Secretariat have ensured communication with the activities of other DRGs and TRGs. However, it was important that the DRG on Zoonoses and other Marginalized Infections (DRG 6) was also in a position, through its expertise and focus in EMRO, to debate the issues in a way that reflected its unique perspective, geographical, health, and livestock and cross-sector experience, since TDR has traditionally not been involved in this group of poverty-promoting infections where interventions span sectors other than health. Although the interaction of most relevance was that with the DRG addressing priorities for helminth diseases (DRG 4), the approaches to control of the zoonotic helminthiases differ significantly from those for non-zoonotic diseases. In addition, DRG 6 felt that more attention should be paid to zoonotic tuberculosis because of the potential importance of bovine tuberculosis in the epidemiology of human tuberculosis in HIV/AIDS patients in Africa. This suggests the need for stronger interactions with the TB DRG (DRG 2) in order to better address research needs in areas where there is evidence of a rate of bovine-derived TB in human cases that is higher than usual.

There are also social science issues relating specifically to the various communities that are livestock-dependent, are not amenable to mainstreaming into society, and traditionally live a migratory and nomadic, pastoralist existence. In this context, a gender perspective is relevant as the roles of the different sexes in these communities are often diverse and traditionally structured. For this reason interventions, on the one hand, and the impact of human and animal diseases, on the other, will have different implications for males and females in these societies. There is a clear relationship also with the TRG addressing environment and agriculture (TRG 4). Environmental and ecological changes will have a profound impact on the diseases covered by TRG 4. Environmental change will lead, for example, to changed migration patterns, potentially increasing contact between livestock-owning communities and settled farming communities (itself a potential source of conflict), which could result in the transmission of infections and outbreaks in farming communities and thus exposure to infections to which people are not traditionally exposed. Environmental change itself, in its many forms, may also result in changes in behaviour and distribution of wildlife reservoir hosts, changed trends in vector or intermediate host biology, and changes in water tables, thus affecting the epidemiology of diseases where aquaculture plays a role (e.g. foodborne trematodes). This subject is an extensive and complex one and will require co-prioritization between DRGs and TRGs. However, as in many settings environmental and ecological change is rapid, constructing and developing research projects that are designed to answer more generic questions is challenging, as many of the issues are often ecologically or geographically specific.

Several sets of health system issues and research questions relate to community interventions (Table 5), i.e. the need for research on interactions at both national and subnational levels between the health sector and those responsible for animal health, as well as other sectors where both human and animal disease research and control can benefit from policy changes, e.g. water and sanitation, wildlife and natural resources. This requires discussion with the Health Systems Group (TRG 3), as it can be anticipated that zoonotic diseases and the specific problems of the livestock-dependent communities, often beyond the end of the road and with no access to the formal health systems, pose specific research questions for these groups.

6.2 Priorities for policy-makers

At present the TDR Stewardship initiative provides possibly the only coordinated global and regional leadership to promote and coordinate an integrated approach to these diseases. As such it represents a model of how this approach may be applied in the context of those communities and ecosystems that facilitate transmission.

The critical factor in progressing the Stewardship agenda consists of moving zoonotic and other marginalized diseases up the research priority agenda while seeking to initiate at-scale implementation of control with known strategies and testing the effectiveness of those strategies against well-monitored baseline data via operational and applied research. However, a prerequisite will be country prioritization and commitment from interested and committed sectors. This approach will require budget lines from both the relevant implementing ministry and national research commitments, stable policy and essential long-term national and international financing.

Promotion of advocacy efforts to inform stakeholders about the societal burden of these diseases is necessary to create demand for control at all levels of society. However, the most serious challenge to overcome is that the diseases to be addressed currently have limited advocacy constituencies and are very often restricted to the most marginalized and disenfranchized communities.

First steps should be to:

- develop guidelines for implementing integrated surveillance to define the problem;
- develop plans for prevention and control activities for these diseases;
- conduct, maintain and report inventories of control activities and tools currently being deployed.

7. Conclusions

The Disease Reference Group focused on zoonoses and marginalized infections. These infections are characteristic of marginalized populations that have little or no access to government services. This may be because of population movement or migration, social or political unrest, conflict, acute natural or human-made disasters provoking complex emergencies, urban populations and slum dwellers, or simply neglect of poor, politically and geographically marginalized populations by the political leadership.

The following research priorities were identified:

- expand the surveillance for zoonotic diseases in humans and animals;
- re-attribute the burden of morbidity and mortality attributed to diseases and conditions (cancers, neurological conditions, injuries) to the neglected parasitic/zoonotic diseases;
- re-evaluate the societal burden of disease for zoonoses;
- expand systems research to determine how best the different sectors can interact;
- evaluate the effectiveness of community-led approaches, including the Community-led Total Sanitation approach, in the control of zoonotic infectious diseases;
- integrate animal and human disease expertise with social science perspectives;
- conduct more extensive studies on the costs of intervention, the cost–benefits and cost–effectiveness;
- scale up research training to increase human resources in the area of public health, including veterinary and livestock services, for addressing zoonoses;
- create opportunities to evaluate and modify control strategies as experience is gained in implementation;
- combine interventions allied to improved water and sanitation, and health education and promotion, and deploy them for the human and animal diseases in parallel;
- expand research on the use of new communication technologies such as smart phones to enhance surveillance, reporting and evaluation.

A need for new scientific discoveries and innovations remains, but a more effective scale-up of existing tools is required across the range of diseases discussed. Effective interventions to address the infections covered do exist but are often not implemented for reasons of cost, lack of policy know-how and the failure to recognize an intervention targeting animals as an alternative approach to reducing the disease burden in humans.

Acknowledgements

Special acknowledgement was made by the DRG to Drs Deborah Kioy, Ayoade Oduola, Johannes Sommerfeld, Lee Willingham, Edith Certain, Julie Reza, and Margaret Harris, Special Programme for Research and Training in Tropical Diseases (TDR), WHO, Geneva, Switzerland, who were instrumental in the creation and management of the DRG as well as the preparation and coordination of the meetings. Valuable support was obtained from Dr Amal Bassili, WHO/EMRO, Cairo, Egypt for the organization and hosting of the stakeholders' consultation.

Support from and contribution made by WHO programmes and staff were valued: Dr François Meslin, Neglected Tropical Diseases, Dr Claire-Lise Chaignat, Water, Sanitation and Hygiene, and Dr Antonio Montresor, Neglected Tropical Diseases, for technical input and participation of meetings. Dr Hind Mohamed Abushama, the TDR Career Development Fellow was involved in the preparation of this report.

The DRG also acknowledged with thanks the valuable contributions made to its work by the stakeholders during the stakeholders' consultation. The stakeholders representing governments: Dr Nasr EL Sayed, Minister's Assistant for Preventive Affairs & Primary Health Care & Family Planning, Ministry of Health, Cairo, Egypt; Dr Fatouh Mostafa Darwish, Head of Central Administration of Preventive Medicine, General Organization for Veterinary Services, Ministry of Agriculture and Land Reclamation, Cairo, Egypt; Dr Hassan Shafik Mohamed, Head of the Central Administration of Public Health and Abattoirs, General Organization for Veterinary Services, Ministry of Agriculture and Land Reclamation, Cairo, Egypt; H.E. Dr Tabita Botrous Shokai, Federal Minister of Health, Federal Ministry of Health, Khartoum, Sudan; H.E. Dr Faysal Hassan Ibrahim, Minister for Animal Resources and Fisheries, Ministry for Animal Resources and Fisheries, Khartoum, Sudan; Dr Sarah Mohamed Awadalla, Director, UN Agencies Directorate, Directorate General of External Relations & International Health, Federal Ministry of Health, Khartoum, Sudan; Dr Nasser Mohsen Baowm, Deputy Minister, Ministry of Public Health and Population, Sana'a, Yemen; Dr Mansoor Mohammed Al Qadasi, Director-General, Animal Health and Veterinary Quarantines, Ministry of Agriculture and Irrigation, Sana'a, Yemen;

Stakeholders representing international and non-governmental organizations: Dr Kathleen Glynn, Chargée de Mission, Scientific and Technical Department, World Organization for Animal Health (OIE), Paris, France; Dr Tarcisse Elongo, Médecin Épidémiologie Provincial, Coordonnateur des Pools de Surveillance, Chef de Sous Bureau de l'OMS au Katanga, Lumbubashi, Congo; Dr Wendy Harrison, Deputy Director, Schistosomiaisis Control Initiative, Department of

Infectious Disease Epidemiology, St Mary's Campus, Norfolk Place, London, England; Dr Aristarchos M. Seimenis, Director, Intercountry Programme, Coordinator WHO/Mediterranean Zoonoses Control Centre, c/o Center of Athens' Veterinary Institutions, Athens, Greece;

Stakeholders representing academic institutions: Professor Samson Mukaratirwa, Head, Biological and Conservation Sciences School, University of KwaZulu-Natal, Durban, South Africa; Dr Esteban Chaves-Olarte, Associate Professor, University of Costa Rica, San José, Costa Rica; Dr Maritza Canales, Academic Coordinator, Masters Program in Infectious and Zoonotic Diseases, School of Microbiology, National Autonomous University of Honduras, Tegucigalpa, Honduras.

Valuable advice and support was received from the members of the informal consultation who helped with the identification of scope for the DRG. These included Dr Vicente Y. Belizario, Jr Deputy Director, National Institutes of Health, and Professor, Department of Parasitology, University of the Philippines, Manila, Philippines; Professor Kirana M. Bhatt, Department of Medicine, College of Health Sciences, University of Nairobi. Kenya; Dr Rosanna Lagos Z. Hospital de Niños Roberto del Río, Santiago, Chile and Dr Nina Mattock, Editor, Bernex, Switzerland.

Sincere thanks and appreciation to the peer reviewers, both from within and outside WHO for their comments and contributions on the technical accuracy of this report. Lisa Nevitt, Centre for Neglected Tropical Diseases, Liverpool School of Tropical Medicine, Liverpool, England, provided support with tables and figures. Dr Philip G. Jenkins was responsible for the technical editing of this report.

The activities of the DRG, including the production of this report, were funded by the Special Programme for Research and Training in Tropical Diseases (TDR) and by European Commission financial support under Agreement PP-AP/2008/160-163.

References

1. Taylor LH, Latham SM, Woolhouse MEJ. Risk factors for human disease emergence. *Philosophical Transactions of the Royal Society of London, Series B*, 2001, 356:983-989.
2. *The control of neglected zoonotic diseases - a route to poverty alleviation. Report of a Joint WHO/ DFID-AHP Meeting with the participation of FAO and OIE*. Geneva, World Health Organization, 2006 (WHO/SDE/FOS/2006.1).
3. Hotez PJ et al. Rescuing the bottom billion through control of neglected tropical diseases. *Lancet*, 2009, 373(9674):1570-1575.
4. Molyneux DH. Combating the "other diseases" of MDG 6: changing the paradigm to achieve equity and poverty reduction? *Transactions of the Royal Society of Tropical Medicine and Hygiene*, 2008, 102(6):509-519.
5. Molyneux DH. Neglected tropical diseases – beyond the tipping point? *Lancet*, 2010, 375(9708): 3-4.
6. Moran M et al. Neglected disease research and development: how much are we really spending? *PLoS Medicine*, 2009, 6(2):30.
7. Liese BL, Schubert L. Official development assistance for health – how neglected are the neglected tropical diseases? An analysis of health financing. *International Health*, 2009, 1(2): 141-147
8. Molyneux D. et al. Zoonoses and marginalised infectious diseases of poverty: Where do we stand? *Parasites & Vectors* 2011, 4:106 http://www.parasitesandvectors.com/content/4/1/106
9 Burke CM, Carabin H, Torgerson PR. Health impact assessment and burden of zoonotic diseases. In: Palmer SR et al., eds. *Oxford textbook of zoonoses: biology, clinical practice, and public health control*. Oxford, Oxford University Press, 2011:30-37.
10. Hyder AA, Morrow RH. Disease burden measurements and trends. In: Merson MH, Black RE, Mills AJ, eds. *International public health. Diseases, programs, systems, and policies*, 2001:1-52.
11. Mathers CD et al. Counting the dead and what they died from: an assessment of the global status of cause of death data. *Bulletin of the World Health Organization*, 2005, 83(3):171-177.
12. Drummond MF et al. Cost-utility analysis. In: *Methods for the economic evaluation of health care programmes*, 3rd ed. Oxford, Oxford University Press, 2005:137-210.
13. Murray CJL, Lopez AD. *The global burden of disease: a comprehensive assessment of mortality and disability from diseases, injuries, and risk factors in 1990 and projected to 2020*. Cambridge, MA, Harvard University Press, 1996.
14. Budke CM, Deplazes P, Torgerson PR. Global socioeconomic impact of cystic echinococcosis. *Emerging Infectious Diseases*, 2006, 12(2):296-303.
15. Knobel DL et al. Re-evaluating the burden of rabies in Africa and Asia. *Bulletin of the World Health Organization*, 2005, 83:360-368.
16. Harrison W. Quantification of the burden of neglected zoonotic diseases in developing countries. In: *Public health in developing countries*. London, London School of Hygiene and Tropical Medicine, 2008.
17. Carabin H et al. Estimation of the cost of *Taenia solium* cysticercosis in Eastern Cape Province, South Africa. *Tropical Medicine and International Health*, 2006, 11(6):906-916.
18. Majorowski MM et al. Echinococcosis in Tunisia: a cost analysis. *Transactions of the Royal Society of Tropical Medicine and Hygiene*, 2005, 99(4):268-278.

19. Acevedo-Hernandez A. *Economic impact of porcine cysticercosis*. In: Flisser A et al., eds. *Cysticercosis: present state of knowledge and perspectives*. New York, Academic Press, 1982:63.
20. Zoli A et al. Regional status, epidemiology and impact of *Taenia solium* cysticercosis in Western and Central Africa. *Acta Tropica*, 2003, 87(1):35-42.
21. Zoli PA, Tchoumboué J. Prevalence de la cysticercose porcine dans le Département de la Menoua (Ouest-Cameroun) [Prevalence of porcine cysticercosis in the department of Menoua (West Cameroon)]. *Cameroon Bulletin of Animal Production*, 1992, 1:42-47.
22. Ito A, Nakao M, Wandra T. Human taeniasis and cysticercosis in Asia. *Lancet*, 2003, 362(9399): 1918-1920.
23. Praet N et al. The annual monetary and disability burden of *Taenia solium* cysticercosis in West Cameroon. *PLOS Neglected Tropical Diseases*, 2009, 3(3):406.
24. Rajkotia Y et al. Economic burden of neurocysticercosis: results from Peru. *Transactions of the Royal Society of Tropical Medicine and Hygiene*, 2007, 101:840-846.
25. Murthy JMK, Rajshekar G. Economic evaluation of seizures associated with solitary cysticercus granuloma. *Neurology India*, 2007, 55:42-45.
26. Croker C, Reporter R, Mascola L. Use of statewide hospital discharge data to evaluate the economic burden of neurocysticercosis in Los Angeles County (1991-2008). *American Journal of Tropical Medicine and Hygiene*, 2010, 83(1):106-110.
27. Torgerson PR, Dowling PM, Abo-Shehada MN. Estimating the economic effects of cystic echinococcosis. Part 3: Jordan, a developing country with lower-middle income. *Annals of Tropical Medicine and Parasitology*, 2001, 95(6):595-603.
28. Torgerson PR, Dowling PM. Estimating the economic effects of cystic echinococcosis. Part 2: an endemic region in the United Kingdom, a wealthy, industrialized economy. *Annals of Tropical Medicine and Parasitology*, 2001, 95(2):177-185.
29. Torgerson PR, Carmona C, Bonifacino R. Estimating the economic effects of cystic echinococcosis: Uruguay, a developing country with upper-middle income. *Annals of Tropical Medicine and Parasitology*, 2000, 94(7):703-713.
30. Budke CM et al. Economic effects of echinococcosis in a disease-endemic region of the Tibetan Plateau. *The American Journal of Tropical Medicine and Hygiene*, 2005, 73(1):2-10.
31. Benner C et al. Analysis of the economic impact of cystic echinococcosis in Spain. *Bulletin of World Health Organization*, 2010, 88(1):49-57.
32. Lembo T et al. The feasibility of canine rabies elimination in Africa: dispelling doubts with data. *PLOS Neglected Tropical Diseases*, 2010, 4(2):626.
33. *WHO Expert Consultation on Rabies. First report*. Geneva, World Health Organization, 2005 (WHO Technical Report Series, No. 931).
34. Hampson K et al. Rabies exposures, post-exposure prophylaxis and deaths in a region of endemic canine rabies. *PLoS Neglected Tropical Diseases*, 2008, 2(11):339.
35. Del Brutto OH et al. Proposed diagnostic criteria for neurocysticercosis. *Neurology*, 2001, 57(2): 177-183.
36. Roman G et al. A proposal to declare neurocysticercosis an international reportable disease. *Bulletin of the World Health Organization*, 2000, 78(3):399-406.
37. Sanchez A, Ljungström I, Medina MT. Diagnosis of human neurocysticercosis in an endemic area: a clinical study in Honduras. *Parasitology International*, 1999, 48:81-89.
38. Ndimubanzi PC et al. A systematic review of the frequency of neurocyticercosis with a focus on people with epilepsy. *PLoS Neglected Tropical Diseases*, 2010, 4(11):870.

39. Puri V et al. Neurocysticercosis in children. *Indian Pediatrics*, 1991, 28(11): 1309-1317.

40. Shasha W, Pammenter MD. Sero-epidemiological studies of cysticercosis in school children from two rural areas of Transkei, South Africa. *Annals of Tropical Medicine and Parasitology*, 1991, 85(3):349-355.

41. Thomson AJG. Neurocysticercosis – experience at the teaching hospitals of the University of Cape Town. *South African Medical Journal*, 1993, 83(5):332-334.

42. Grill J et al. High prevalence of serological markers of cysticercosis among epileptic Malagasy children. *Annals of Tropical Paediatrics*, 1996, 16(3):185-191.

43. Rosenfeld EA, Byrd SE, Shulman ST. Neurocysticercosis among children in Chicago. *Clinical Infectious Diseases*, 1996, 23(2):262-268.

44. Talukdar B et al. Neurocysticercosis in children: clinical characteristics and outcome. *Annals of Tropical Paediatrics*, 2002, 22(4):333-339.

45. Mafojane NA et al. The current status of neurocysticercosis in Eastern and Southern Africa. *Acta Tropica*, 2003, 87(1):25-33.

46. Gaffo AL et al. [Cysticercosis as the main cause of partial seizures in children in Peru]. *Revista de Neurologia*, 2004, 39(10):924-926.

47. Carabin H et al. Monetary burden of *Taenia solium* cysticercosis in Honduras, India, and South Africa. In: *Annual Meeting & Exposition*, Philadelphia, PA, USA, American Public Health Association, 2005:10-14.

48. Recommendations of the International Task Force for Disease Eradication. *MMWR Recommendations and Reports*, 1993, 42(RR-16):1-38.

49. ITFDE and I.T.F.f.D.E. II., *Summary of the Fourth Meeting of the ITFDE (II)*, 2003.

50. *Global plan to combat neglected tropical diseases 2008-2015*. Geneva, World Health Organization, 2007 (WHO/CDS/NTD/2007.3).

51. *Integrated control of neglected zoonotic diseases in Africa: applying the one health concept. Report of a joint WHO/EU/ILRI/ DBL/FAO/OIE/AU meeting, ILRI headquarters, Nairobi, 13-15 November 2007*. Geneva, World Health Organization, 2009 (WHO/HTM/NTD/NZD/2008.1).

52. *The global burden of foodborne diseases: taking stock and charting the way forward. WHO Consultation to Develop a Strategy to Estimate the Global Burden of Foodborne Diseases, Geneva, 25-27 September 2006*. Geneva, World Health Organization, 2006.

53. *First formal meeting of the Foodborne Disease Burden Epidemiology Reference Group (FERG): implementing strategy, setting priorities and assigning the tasks*. Geneva, World Health Organization, 2007.

54. *Second formal meeting of the Foodborne Disease Burden Epidemiology Reference Group (FERG): appraising the evidence and reviewing initial results*. Geneva, World Health Organization, 2008.

55. Willingham AL, Mugarura A. *Taenia solium* tapeworms and epilepsy in Uganda. *International Epilepsy News*, 2008(1):10-12.

56. Zhou XN et al. RNAS(+): A win-win collaboration to combat neglected tropical diseases in Southeast Asia. *Parasitology International*, 2008, 57(3):243-245.

57. Willingham AL IIIrd et al. Inaugural meeting of the Cysticercosis Working Group in Europe. *Emerging Infectious Diseases*, 2008, 14(12):2.

58. Murrell KD. *WHO/FAO/OIE Guidelines for the surveillance, prevention and control of taeniosis/cysticercosis*. Paris, Office International des Epizooties, 2005.

59. Garcia HH et al. Combined human and porcine mass chemotherapy for the control of *T. solium*. *The American Journal of Tropical Medicine and Hygiene*, 2006, 74(5):850-855.

60. Ngowi HA et al. A health-education intervention trial to reduce porcine cysticercosis in Mbulu District, Tanzania. *Preventive Veterinary Medicine*, 2008, 85(1-2):52-67.

61. Kyvsgaard NC, Johansen MV, H. Carabin. Simulating transmission and control of *Taenia solium* infections using a Reed-Frost stochastic model. *International Journal of Parasitology*, 2007, 37(5):547-58.

62. Caulfield LE et al. Undernutrition as an underlying cause of child deaths associated with diarrhea, pneumonia, malaria, and measles. *The American Journal of Clinical Nutrition*, 2004, 80(1):193-198.

63. Brandt JR et al. A monoclonal antibody-based ELISA for the detection of circulating excretory-secretory antigens in *Taenia saginata* cysticercosis. *International Journal of Parasitology*, 1992, 22(4):471-417.

64. Thomas SV et al. Economic burden of epilepsy in India. *Epilepsia*, 2001, 42(8):1052-1060.

65. Boa ME et al. Distribution and density of cysticerci of *Taenia solium* by muscle groups and organs in naturally infected local finished pigs in Tanzania. *Veterinary Parasitology*, 2002, 106(2):155-164.

66. Carpio A. Neurocysticercosis: an update. *The Lancet Infectious Diseases*, 2002, 2(12):751-762.

67. Carpio A, Hauser WA. Prognosis for seizure recurrence in patients with newly diagnosed neurocysticercosis. *Neurology*, 2002, 59(11):1730-1734.

68. Avode DG et al. [Epilepsy caused by cysticercosis. A propos of a sociological and cultural investigation conducted at Savalou in Benin]. *Bulletin de la Société de Pathologie exotique et de ses Fillales*, 1996, 89(1):45-7.

69. Preux PM et al. Antiepileptic therapies in the Mifi Province in Cameroon. *Epilepsia*, 2000, 41(4):432-439.

70. Birbeck G et al. The social and economic impact of epilepsy in Zambia: a cross-sectional study. *Lancet Neurology*, 2007, 6(1):39-44.

71. Carabin H et al. Assessing the infection burden of cysticercosis and echinococcosis. *Trends in Parasitology*, 2005, 21:327-333.

72. Praet N et al. The disease burden of *Taenia solium* cysticercosis in Cameroon. *PLoS Neglected Tropical Diseases*, 2009, 3(3):406.

73. Jenkins DJ, Romig T, Thompson RC. Emergence/re-emergence of *Echinococcus* spp: a global update. *International Journal of Parasitology*, 2005, 35(11-12):1205-1219.

74. Brunetti E, Kern P, Vuitton DA. Expert consensus for the diagnosis and treatment of cystic and alveolar echinococcosis in humans. *Acta Tropica*, 2010, 114(1):1-16.

75. Torgerson PR et al. The global burden of alveolar echinococcosis. *PLoS Neglected Tropical Diseases*, 2010, 4(6):722.

76. Craig PS, Larrieu E, Control of cystic echinococcosis/hydatidosis: 1863-2002. *Advances in Parasitology*, 2006, 61:443-508.

77. Chen MG. *Schistosoma japonicum* and *S. japonicum*-like infections – epidemiology, clinical and pathological aspects. In: Jordan P et al., eds. *Human schistosomisis*. Oxford, CAB International, 1993:242-243.

78. Carabin H et al. Estimating sensitivity and specificity of a faecal examination method for *Schistosoma japonicum* infection in cats, dogs, water buffaloes, pigs, and rats in Western Samar and Sorsogon Provinces, The Philippines. *International Journal of Parasitology*, 2005, 35(14):1517-1524.

79. Wang TP et al. Transmission of *Schistosoma japonicum* by humans and domestic animals in the Yangtze River valley, Anhui province, China. *Acta Tropica*, 2005, 96(2-3):198-204.

80. Wang T et al. Treatment and reinfection of water buffaloes and cattle infected with *Schistosoma japonicum* in Yangtze River Valley, Anhui province, China. *The Journal of Parasitology*, 2006, 92(5):1088-1091.

81. McManus DP et al. Schistosomiasis in the People's Republic of China: the era of the Three Gorges Dam. *Clinical Microbiology Reviews*, 2010, 23(2):442-466.

82. Finkelstein JL et al. Decision-model estimation of the age-specific disability weight for *Schistosoma japonicum*: a systematic review of the literature. *PLoS Neglected Tropical Diseases*, 2008, 2(3):158.

83. McGarvey ST et al. Cross-sectional associations between intensity of animal and human infection with *Schistosoma japonicum* in Western Samar province, Philippines. *Bulletin of the World Health Organization*, 2006, 84(6):446-452.

84. Wu HW et al. High prevalence of *Schistosoma japonicum* infection in water buffaloes in the Philippines assessed by real-time polymerase chain reaction. *The American Journal of Tropical Medicine and Hygiene*, 2010, 82(4):646-652.

85. Sinuon M et al. Control of *Schistosoma mekongi* in Cambodia: results of eight years of control activities in the two endemic provinces. *Transactions of the Royal Society of Tropical Medicine and Hygiene*, 2007, 101(1):34-39.

86. Wu WH et al. The process and strategy in elimination of schistosomiasis in Guangdong, Shanghai, Fujian, Guangxi, Zhejiang provinces. In: Wang LD, ed. *The course and perspectives in schistosomiasis control in China*. Beijing, People's Health Press, 2006:401.

87. Leonardo LR et al. Difficulties and strategies in the control of schistosomiasis in the Philippines. *Acta Tropica*, 2002, 82(2):295-299.

88. Tallo VL et al. Is mass treatment the appropriate schistosomiasis elimination strategy? *Bulletin of the World Health Organization*, 2008, 86(10):765-771.

89. Wang LD et al. A strategy to control transmission of *Schistosoma japonicum* in China. *The New England Journal of Medicine*, 2009, 360(2):121-128.

90. Utzinger J et al. Conquering schistosomiasis in China: the long march. *Acta Tropica*, 2005, 96(2-3):69-96.

91. McManus DP, Loukas A. Current status of vaccines for schistosomiasis. *Clinical Microbiology Reviews*, 2008, 21(1):225-42.

92. Zhu HM et al. Three Gorges Dam and its impact on the potential transmission of schistosomiasis in regions along the Yangtze River. *Ecohealth*, 2008, 5(2):137-148.

93. Croce D et al. Cost-effectiveness of a successful schistosomiasis control programme in Cambodia (1995-2006). *Acta Tropica*, 2010, 113(3):279-84.

94. Keiser J, Utzinger J. Food-borne trematodiases. *Clinical Microbiology Reviews*, 2009, 22(3):466-483.

95. Sripa B et al. Liver fluke induces cholangiocarcinoma. PLoS Medicine, 2007, 4(7):201.

96. Sripa B. Pathobiology of opisthorchiasis: an update. *Acta Tropica*, 2003, 88(3):209-220.

97. Mas-Coma S, Bargues MD, Valero MA. Fascioliasis and other plant-borne trematode zoonoses. *International Journal of Parasitology*, 2005, 35(11-12):1255-1278.

98. Phan VT et al. Farm-level risk factors for fish-borne zoonotic trematode infection in integrated small-scale fish farms in northern Vietnam. *PLoS Neglected Tropical Diseases*, 2010, 4(7):742.

99. *Report: Joint WHO/FAO Workshop on Foodborne Trematode Infections in Asia, Hanoi, Viet Nam, 26-28 Novermber 2002*. Geneva, World Health Organization, 2004.

100. Keiser J, Utzinger J. Emerging foodborne trematodiasis. *Emerging Infectious Diseases*, 2005, 11(10):1507-1514.

101. Remington JS et al. *Toxoplasmosis. In:* Remington JS et al. *eds. Infectious diseases of the fetus and newborn infant. 6th ed. Philadelphia: Elsevier Saunders; 2006. p. 947-1091.*

102. Rosso F et al. Progress in science and action. In: *International Conference on Women and Infectious Diseases*. GA, Atlanta, 2006.

103. CDC. Cryptosporidiosis: assessment of chemotherapy of males with acquired immune deficiency syndrome (AIDS). *MMWR Morbidity and Mortality Weekly Report*, 1982, 31(44):589-92.

104. Xiao L, Fayer R. Molecular characterisation of species and genotypes of *Cryptosporidium* and *Giardia* and assessment of zoonotic transmission. *International Journal of Parasitology*, 2008, 38(11):1239-1255.

105. McLauchlin J et al. Molecular epidemiological analysis of *Cryptosporidium* spp. in the United Kingdom: results of genotyping *Cryptosporidium* spp. in 1,705 fecal samples from humans and 105 fecal samples from livestock animals. *Journal of Clinical Microbiology*, 2000, 38(11):3984-3990.

106. Feltus DC et al. Evidence supporting zoonotic transmission of *Cryptosporidium* spp. in Wisconsin. *Journal of Clinical Microbiology*, 2006, 44(12):4303-4308.

107. Smith KE et al. Outbreaks of enteric infections caused by multiple pathogens associated with calves at a farm day camp. *The Pediatric Infectious Disease Journal*, 2004, 23(12):1098-1104.

108. Kiang KM et al. Recurrent outbreaks of cryptosporidiosis associated with calves among students at an educational farm programme, Minnesota, 2003. *Epidemiology and Infection*, 2006, 134(4):878-86.

109. Pohjola S et al. Outbreak of cryptosporidiosis among veterinary students. *Scandinavian Journal of Infectious Diseases*, 1986, 18(2):173-178.

110. Tzipori S. Cryptosporidiosis in animals and humans. *Microbiological Reviews*, 1983, 47(1):84-96.

111. Miao YM et al. Eradication of cryptosporidia and microsporidia following successful antiretroviral therapy. *Journal of Acquired Immune Deficiency Syndrome*, 2000, 25(2):124-129.

112. Wolfson JS et al. Cryptosporidiosis in immunocompetent patients. *New England Journal of Medicine*, 1985, 312(20):1278-1282.

113. DuPont HL et al. The infectivity of *Cryptosporidium parvum* in healthy volunteers. *New England Journal of Medicine*, 1995. 332(13):855-859.

114. Mac Kenzie WR et al. A massive outbreak in Milwaukee of cryptosporidium infection transmitted through the public water supply. *New England Journal of Medicine*, 1994, 331(3):161-167.

115. Frisby HR et al. Clinical and epidemiologic features of a massive waterborne outbreak of cryptosporidiosis in persons with HIV infection. *Journal of Acquired Immune Deficiency Syndromes and Human Retrovirology*, 1997, 16(5):367-373.

116. Kaplan JE et al. Epidemiology of human immunodeficiency virus-associated opportunistic infections in the United States in the era of highly active antiretroviral therapy. *Clinical Infrectious Diseases*, 2000, 30(Suppl 1):5-14.

117. Corso PS et al. Cost of illness in the 1993 waterborne Cryptosporidium outbreak, Milwaukee, Wisconsin. *Emerging Infectious Diseases*, 2003, 9(4):426-431.

118. Yoder JS, Beach MJ. Cryptosporidium surveillance and risk factors in the United States. *Experimental Parasitology*, 2010, 124(1):31-39.

119. Mor SM, Tzipori S. Cryptosporidiosis in children in sub-Saharan Africa: a lingering challenge. *Clinical Infectious Diseases*, 2008, 47(7):915-921.

120. Perch M et al. Seven years' experience with *Cryptosporidium parvum* in Guinea-Bissau, West Africa. *Annals of Tropical Paediatrics*, 2001, 21(4):313-318.

121. Valentiner-Branth P et al. Cohort study of Guinean children: incidence, pathogenicity, conferred protection, and attributable risk for enteropathogens during the first 2 years of life. *Journal of Clinical Microbiology*, 2003, 41(9):4238-4245.

122. Gatei W et al. Cryptosporidiosis: prevalence, genotype analysis, and symptoms associated with infections in children in Kenya. *The American Journal of Tropical Medicine and Hygiene*, 2006, 75(1):78-82.

123. Morse TD et al. Incidence of cryptosporidiosis species in paediatric patients in Malawi. *Epidemiology and Infection*, 2007, 135(8):1307-1315.

124. Robinson TJ et al. Evaluation of the positive predictive value of rapid assays used by clinical laboratories in Minnesota for the diagnosis of cryptosporidiosis. *Clinical Infectious Diseases*, 2010, 50(8):53-5.

125. Jokipii L, Jokipii AM. Timing of symptoms and oocyst excretion in human cryptosporidiosis. *New England Journal of Medicine*, 1986, 315(26):1643-1647.

126. Rossignol JF. *Cryptosporidium* and *Giardia*: treatment options and prospects for new drugs. *Experimental Parasitology*, 2010, 124(1):45-53.

127. Amadi B et al. High dose prolonged treatment with nitazoxanide is not effective for cryptosporidiosis in HIV positive Zambian children: a randomised controlled trial. *BMC Infectious Diseases*, 2009, 9:195.

128. de Graaf DC et al. A review of the importance of cryptosporidiosis in farm animals. *International Journal of Parasitology*, 1999, 29(8):1269-1287.

129. Harp JA, Goff JP. Strategies for the control of *Cryptosporidium parvum* infection in calves. *Journal of Dairy Science*, 1998, 81(1):289-294.

130. Moreno E, Moreno MI. The genus *Brucella*. In: Dworkin M et al., eds *The prokaryotes, Vol. 5*, 3rd ed. New York, Springer-Verlag, 2006:315-456.

131. Clavareau C et al. Phenotypic and molecular characterization of a *Brucella* strain isolated from a minke whale (*Balaenoptera acutorostrata*). *Microbiology*, 1998, 144(12):3267-3273.

132. Zribi M et al. [Clinical manifestations, complications and treatment of brucellosis: 45-patient study]. *Pathologie - Biologie*, 2009, 57(5):349-352.

133. Thakur SD, Kumar R, Thapliyal DC. Human brucellosis: review of an under-diagnosed animal transmitted disease. *Journal of Communicable Diseases*, 2002, 34(4):287-301.

134. Reyburn H et al. Overdiagnosis of malaria in patients with severe febrile illness in Tanzania: a prospective study. *British Medical Journal*, 2004, 329(7476):1212

135. John K, Kazwala R, Mfinanga GS. Knowledge of causes, clinical features and diagnosis of common zoonoses among medical practitioners in Tanzania. *BMC Infectious Diseases*, 2008, 8:162.

136. Cutler SJ, Whatmore AM, Commander NJ. Brucellosis: new aspects of an old disease. *Journal of Applied Microbiology*, 2005, 98(6):1270-1281.

137. Kunda J et al. Health-seeking behaviour of human brucellosis cases in rural Tanzania. *BMC Public Health*, 2007, 7:315.

138. McDermott JJ, Arimi SM. Brucellosis in sub-Saharan Africa: epidemiology, control and impact. *Veterinary Microbiology*, 2002, 90(1-4):111-134.

139. Kunda, J. *Epidemiology of zoonoses in the context of brucellosis in Tanzania.*, Edinburgh, University of Edinburgh, 2007.

140. Keusch GT et al. Diarrheal diseases. In: Jamison DT et al., eds. *Disease control priorities in developing countries*. Oxford, Oxford University Press, 2006:371-387.

141. Ochoa TJ, Salazar-Lindo E, Cleary TG. Management of children with infection-associated persistent diarrhea. *Seminars in Pediatric Infectious Diseases*, 2004, 15(4):229-236.

142. Keusch GT. Shigellosis. In: Brachman PS, Abrutyn E, eds. *Bacterial infections of humans*, New York, Plenum Press, 2009.

143. Raqib R et al. Persistence of local cytokine production in shigellosis in acute and convalescent stages. *Infection and Immunity*, 1995, 63(1):289-296.

144. Keusch GT, Scrimshaw NS. Selective primary health care: strategies for control of disease in the developing world. XXIII. Control of infection to reduce the prevalence of infantile and childhood malnutrition. *Reviews of Infectious Diseases*, 1986, 8(2):273-287.

145. Bejon P et al. Fraction of all hospital admissions and deaths attributable to malnutrition among children in rural Kenya. *American Journal of Clinical Nutrition*, 2008, 88(6):1626-1631.

146. Scrimshaw NS, Taylor CE, Gordon JE. Interactions of nutrition and infection. *American Journal of the Medical Sciences*, 1959, 237(3):367-403.

147. Boschi-Pinto CL, Velebit, Shibuya K. Estimating child mortality due to diarrhoea in developing countries. *Bulletin of the World Health Organization*, 2008, 86(9):710-717.

148. Petri WA et al. Enteric infections, diarrhea, and their impact on function and development. *Journal of Clinical Investigation*, 2008. 118(4):1277-1290.

149. Kotloff KL et al. Global burden of *Shigella* infections: implications for vaccine development and implementation of control strategies. *Bulletin of the World Health Organization*, 1999, 77(8):651-666.

150. Snyder JD, Merson MH. The magnitude of the global problem of acute diarrhoeal disease: a review of active surveillance data. *Bulletin of the World Health Organization*, 1982, 60(4):605-613.

151. Bern C et al. The magnitude of the global problem of diarrhoeal disease: a ten-year update. *Bulletin of the World Health Organization*, 1992, 70(6):705-714.

152. Kosek M, Bern C, Guerrant RL. The global burden of diarrhoeal disease, as estimated from studies published between 1992 and 2000. *Bulletin of the World Health Organization*, 2003, 81(3):197-204.

153. Parashar UD, Bresee JS, Glass RI. The global burden of diarrhoeal disease in children. *Bulletin of the World Health Organization*, 2003, 81(4):236.

154. The global burden of disease: 2004 update. Geneva, World Health Organization, 2008.

155. Cholera: global surveillance summary, 2008. *Weekly Epidemiological Record*, 2009, 84(31):309-324.

156. Kanungo S et al. Cholera in India: an analysis of reports, 1997-2006. *Bulletin of the World Health Organization*, 2010, 88(3):185-191.

157. Tiruneh M. Serodiversity and antimicrobial resistance pattern of *Shigella* isolates at Gondar University teaching hospital, Northwest Ethiopia. *Japanese Journal of Infectious Diseases*, 2009, 62(2):93-97.

158. Kerneis S et al. A look back at an ongoing problem: *Shigella dysenteriae* type 1 epidemics in refugee settings in Central Africa (1993-1995). *PLoS One*, 2009, 4(2):4494.

159. Connolly MA et al. Communicable diseases in complex emergencies: impact and challenges. *Lancet*, 2004, 364(9449):1974-1983.

160. Bollet AJ. The major infectious epidemic diseases of Civil War soldiers. *Infectious Diseases Clinics of North America*, 2004, 18(2):293-309.

161. Chastel C. [The centenary of the discovery of the vibrio El Tor (1905) or dubious beginnings of the seventh pandemic of cholera]. *Histoire des Sciences Médicales*, 2007, 41(1):71-82.

162. Pollitzer R. Cholera studies. 1. History of the disease. *Bulletin of the World Health Organization*, 1954, 10(3):421-461.

163. Ahmed QA, Arabi YM, Memish ZA. Health risks at the Hajj. *Lancet*, 2006, 367(9515):1008-1015.

164. Mead PS et al. Food-related illness and death in the United States. *Emerging Infectious Diseases*, 1999, 5(5):607-625.

165. Scharff RL. *Health-related costs from foodborne illness in the United States*. Washington, DC. Produce Safety Project at Georgetown University, 2010.

166. Keusch GT et al., eds. *Institute of Medicine and National Research Council, Sustaining Global surveillance and response to emerging zoonotic diseases*. Washington DC, The National Academic Press, 2009.

167. WHO. *Seven neglected endemic zoonoses - some basic facts*. World Health Organization, 2009.

168. O'Reilly LM, Daborn CJ. The epidemiology of *Mycobacterium bovis* infections in animals and man: a review. *Tubercle and lung disease*, 1995, 76(Suppl 1):1-46.

169. Cosivi O et al. Zoonotic tuberculosis due to *Mycobacterium bovis* in developing countries. *Emerging Infectious Diseases*, 1998, 4(1):59-70.

170. Grange JM. *Mycobacterium bovis* infection in human beings. *Tuberculosis (Edinburgh, Scotland)*, 2001, 81(1-2):71-77.

171. Michel AL, Muller B, van Helden PD. *Mycobacterium bovis* at the animal-human interface: a problem, or not? *Veterinary Microbiology*, 2010, 140(3-4):371-381.

172. Marcotty T et al. Zoonotic tuberculosis and brucellosis in Africa: neglected zoonoses or minor public-health issues? The outcomes of a multi-disciplinary workshop. *Annals of Tropical Medicine and Parasitology*, 2009, 103(5):401-411.

173. Cadmus S et al. Molecular analysis of human and bovine tubercle bacilli from a local setting in Nigeria. *Journal of Clinical Microbiology*, 2006, 44(1):29-34.

174. Kazwala RR et al. Isolation of *Mycobacterium bovis* from human cases of cervical adenitis in Tanzania: a cause for concern? *International Journal of Tuberculosis and Lung Disease*, 2001, 5(1):87-91.

175. Mfinanga SG et al. Mycobacterial adenitis: role of *Mycobacterium bovis*, non-tuberculous mycobacteria, HIV infection, and risk factors in Arusha, Tanzania. *East African Medical Journal*, 2004, 81(4):171-178.

176. Oloya J et al. Mycobacteria causing human cervical lymphadenitis in pastoral communities in the Karamoja region of Uganda. *Epidemiology and Infection*, 2008, 136(5):636-643.

177. Byarugaba F et al. Pulmonary tuberculosis and *Mycobacterium bovis*, Uganda. *Emerging Infectious Diseases*, 2009, 15(1):124-125.

178. Jou R, Huang WL, Chiang CY. Human tuberculosis caused by *Mycobacterium bovis, Taiwan Emerging Infectious Diseases*, 2008, 14(3):515-517.

179. Coleman P. Zoonotic diseases and their impact on the poor. In: Perry BD et al., eds. *Investing in animal health research to alleviate poverty*. Kenya, Nairobi, International Livestock Research Institute 2002.

180. Cleaveland S et al. *Mycobacterium bovis* in rural Tanzania: risk factors for infection in human and cattle populations. *Tuberculosis (Edinburg, Scotland)*, 2007, 87(1):30-43.

181. Jindal N, Devi B, Aggarwal A. Mycobacterial cervical lymphadenitis in childhood. *Indian Journal of Medical Sciences*, 2003, 57(1):12-15.

182. Perry BD et al. *Investing in animal health research to alleviate poverty*. Nairobi, International Livestock Research Institute, 2002.

183. WHO. *WHO Expert Consultation on Rabies: First Report*. Geneva, World Health Organization, 2004.
184. Coleman PG, Dye C. Immunization coverage required to prevent outbreaks of dog rabies. *Vaccine*, 1996, 14(3):185-186.
185. Cleaveland S et al. A dog rabies vaccination campaign in rural Africa: impact on the incidence of dog rabies and human dog-bite injuries. *Vaccine*, 2003, 21(17-18):1965-1973.
186. Hampson K et al. Transmission dynamics and prospects for the elimination of canine rabies. *PLoS Biology*, 2009, 7(3):53.
187. Sudarshan MK et al. Assessing the burden of human rabies in India: results of a national multi-center epidemiological survey. *International Journal of Infectious Diseases*, 2007, 11(1):29-35.
188. Schneider MC et al. Current status of human rabies transmitted by dogs in Latin America. *Cadernos de saúde pública*, 2007, 23(9):2049-2063.
189. Hodgkin C et al. The future of onchocerciasis control in Africa. *PLoS Neglected Tropical Diseases*, 2007, 1(1):74.
190. Homeida M et al. APOC's strategy of community-directed treatment with ivermectin (CDTI) and its potential for providing additional health services to the poorest populations. African Programme for Onchocerciasis Control. *Annals of Tropical Medicine and Parasitology*, 2002, 96(Suppl 1):93-104.
191. CDI. Community-directed interventions for priority health problems in Africa: results of a multicountry study. *Bulletin of the World Health Organization*, 2010, 88(7):509-518.
192. Cairncross S. Health impacts in developing countries: new evidence and new prospects. *Journal of the Institution of Water and Environmental Managemen*t, 1990, 4:571–577.
193. Strina A et al. Childhood diarrhea and observed hygiene behavior in Salvador, Brazil. *American Journal of Epidemiology*, 2003, 157(11):1032-1038.
194. Ferrer SR et al. A hierarchical model for studying risk factors for childhood diarrhoea: a case-control study in a middle-income country. *International Journal of Epidemiology*, 2008, 37(4):805-815.
195. Genser B et al. Impact of a city-wide sanitation intervention in a large urban centre on social, environmental and behavioural determinants of childhood diarrhoea: analysis of two cohort studies. *International Journal of Epidemiology*, 2008, 37(4):831-840.
196. Cairncross S et al. Water, sanitation and hygiene for the prevention of diarrhoea. *International Journal of Epidemiology*, 2010, 39(Suppl 1):193-205.
197. Kar K, Chambers R. *Handbook on community-led total sanitation*. London, Plan International, 2008.
198. Clasen TF et al. Interventions to improve disposal of human excreta for preventing diarrhoea. *Cochrane Database of Systematic Reviews*, 2010, 6:CD007180.
199. *Preventive chemotherapy in human helminthiasis. Coordinated use of antihelminthic drugs in control interventions: a manual for health professionals and programme managers*. Geneva, World Health Organization, 2006.
200. *Control of foodborne trematode infections. Report of a WHO Study Group*. Geneva, World Health Organization, 1995 (WHO Technical Report Series, No. 849).
201. Gabriella F et al., Food borne trematode (FBT) infections : WHO/NTD's position. *PLoS Neglected Tropical Deseases Correspondence*, 2008.
202. Fenwick A, Rollinson D, Southgate V. Implementation of human schistosomiasis control: challenges and prospects. *Advances in Parasitology*, 2006, 61:567-622.

203. Flisser A, Craig PS. Larval cestodes in parasitology. In: Cox FEG et al., eds. *Topley and Wilson's microbiology and microbial infections*, 10th ed. London, Arnold, 2005.

204. Gemmell MA, Roberts MG. Cystic echinococcosis (*Echinococcus granulosus*). In: Palmer SR, Lord Soulsby, Simpson DIH, eds. Zoonoses. Oxford, Oxford University Press, 1998:665-688.

205. Assana E et al. Elimination of *Taenia solium* transmission to pigs in a field trial of the TSOL18 vaccine in Cameroon. *International Journal for Parasitology*, 2010, 40(5):515-519.

206. Periago MR et al. Elimination of cholera transmission in Haiti and the Dominican Republic. *Lancet*, 2012; 379(9812):e12-13.

207. McCullough FS. Snail control in relation to a strategy for reduction of morbidity due to schistosomiasis. *Tropical Medicine and Parasitology*, 1986, 37(2):181-184.

208. Gundersen SG et al. Control of *Schistosoma mansoni* in the Blue Nile Valley of western Ethiopia by mass chemotherapy and focal snail control: a primary health care experience. *Transactions of the Royal Society of Tropical Medicine and Hygiene*, 1990, 84(6):819-825.

209. Umeno S, Doi Y. A study on the anti-rabic inoculation of dogs and the results of its practical application. *The Kitasato Archives of Experimental Medicine* 1921, (4):89–108

210. Steck F et al. Oral immunization of foxes against rabies. Laboratory and field studies. *Comparative Immunology, Microbiology and Infectious Diseases*, 1982, 5(1-3):165-171.

211. Gray DJ et al. Transmission dynamics of *Schistosoma japonicum* in the lakes and marshlands of China. *PLoS One*, 2008, 3(12):4058.

212. Da'dara AA et al. DNA-based vaccines protect against zoonotic schistosomiasis in water buffalo. *Vaccine*, 2008, 26(29-30):3617-3625.

213. Williams GM et al. Mathematical modelling of *Schistosomiasis japonica*: comparison of control strategies in the People's Republic of China. *Acta Tropica*, 2002, 82(2):253-262.

214. Berriman M et al. The genome of the blood fluke *Schistosoma mansoni*. *Nature*, 2009, 460(7253):352-358.

215. The *Schistosoma japonicum* genome reveals features of host-parasite interplay. *Nature*, 2009, 460(7253):345-351.

216. Lightowlers MW. Vaccines against cysticercosis and hydatidosis: foundations in taeniid cestode immunology. *Parasitoogy International*, 2006, 55(Suppl):39-43.

217. Craig PS et al. Prevention and control of cystic echinococcosis. *Lancet Infectious Disease*, 2007, 7(6):385-394.

218. Zhang W et al. Vaccination of dogs against *Echinococcus granulosus*, the cause of cystic hydatid disease in humans. *Journal of Infectious Diseases*, 2006, 194(7):966-974.

219. Petavy AF et al. An oral recombinant vaccine in dogs against *Echinococcus granulosus*, the causative agent of human hydatid disease: a pilot study. *PLoS Neglected Tropical Diseases*, 2008, 2(1):125.

220. Torgerson PR. Dogs, vaccines and *Echinococcus*. *Trends in Parasitology*, 2009, 25(2):57-58.

221. Lightowlers MW. Eradication of *Taenia solium* cysticercosis: a role for vaccination of pigs. *International Journal for Parasitology*, 2010, 40(10):1183-1192.

222. McManus DP, Dalton JP. Vaccines against the zoonotic trematodes *Schistosoma japonicum*, *Fasciola hepatica* and *Fasciola gigantica*. *Parasitology*, 2006, 133(Suppl):43-61.

223. Jayaraj R et al., Vaccination against fasciolosis by a multivalent vaccine of stage-specific antigens. *Veterinary Parasitology*, 2009, 160(3-4):230-236.

224. Madhi SA et al., Effect of human rotavirus vaccine on severe diarrhea in African infants. *New England Journal of Medicine*, 2010, 362(4):289-298.

225. Santosham M. Rotavirus vaccine – a powerful tool to combat deaths from diarrhea. *New England Journal of Medicine*, 2010, 362(4):358-360.

226. Patel M et al. Oral rotavirus vaccines: how well will they work where they are needed most? *Journal of Infectious Diseases*, 2009, 200(Suppl 1):39-48.

227. Fu C et al. Effectiveness of Lanzhou lamb rotavirus vaccine against rotavirus gastroenteritis requiring hospitalization: a matched case-control study. *Vaccine*, 2007, 25(52):8756-8761.

228. Lopez AL et al. Cholera vaccines for the developing world. *Human Vaccines*, 2008, 4(2):165-169.

229. Trach DD et al. Field trial of a locally produced, killed, oral cholera vaccine in Vietnam. *Lancet*, 1997, 349(9047):231-235.

230. Anh DD et al. Safety and immunogenicity of a reformulated Vietnamese bivalent killed, whole-cell, oral cholera vaccine in adults. *Vaccine*, 2007, 25(6): 1149-1155.

231. Sur D et al. Efficacy and safety of a modified killed-whole-cell oral cholera vaccine in India: an interim analysis of a cluster-randomised, double-blind, placebo-controlled trial. *Lancet*, 2009, 374(9702):1694-1702.

232. *WHO Cholera*, in *World Health Organization*. Geneva, World Health Organization, 2010.

233. Phalipon A, Mulard LA, Sansonetti PJ. Vaccination against shigellosis: is it the path that is difficult or is it the difficult that is the path? *Microbes and Infection* 2008, 10(9):1057-1062.

234. Launay O et al. Safety and immunogenicity of SC599, an oral live attenuated *Shigella dysenteriae* type-1 vaccine in healthy volunteers: results of a Phase 2, randomized, double-blind placebo-controlled trial. *Vaccine*, 2009, 27(8):1184-1891.

235. Xu de Q et al. Core-linked LPS expression of *Shigella dysenteriae* serotype 1 O-antigen in live *Salmonella typhi* vaccine vector Ty21a: preclinical evidence of immunogenicity and protection. *Vaccine*, 2007, 25(33):6167-675.

236. Turbyfill KR, Hartman AB, Oaks EV. Isolation and characterization of a *Shigella flexneri* invasin complex subunit vaccine. *Infection and Immunity*, 2000, 68(12):6624-6632.

237. Cohen D et al. Double-blind vaccine-controlled randomised efficacy trial of an investigational *Shigella sonnei* conjugate vaccine in young adults. *Lancet*, 1997, 349(9046):155-159.

238. Levine MM et al. Clinical trials of Shigella vaccines: two steps forward and one step back on a long, hard road. *Nature Reviews. Microbiology*, 2007, 5(7):540-553.

239. Fevre EM et al. Human African trypanosomiasis: epidemiology and control. *Advances in Parasitology*, 2006, 61:167-221.

240. Hotez PJ et al. Control of neglected tropical diseases. *New England Journal of Medicine*, 2007, 357(10):1018-1027.

241. Cutler DM, Lleras-Muney A. Understanding differences in health behaviors by education. *Journal of Health Economics*, 2009, 29(1):1-28.

242. *Toward universal primary education: investments, incentives, and institutions*. New York, UN Millennium Project, 2005:207.

243. *Achieving health equity: from root causes to fair outcomes. Commission on Social Determinants of Health: interim statement*. Geneva, World Health Organization, 2007.

244. Sanchez AL, Medina MT, Ljungstrom I. Prevalence of taeniasis and cysticercosis in a population of urban residence in Honduras. *Acta Tropica*, 1998, 69(2):141-149.

245. Moro PL et al. *Taenia solium* infection in a rural community in the Peruvian Andes. *Annals of Tropical Medicine and Parasitology*, 2003, 97(4):373-379.

246. Huang YX, Manderson L. The social and economic context and determinants of *Schistosomiasis japonica*. *Acta Tropica*, 2005, 96(2-3):223-231.

247. Sarti E et al. Development and evaluation of a health education intervention against *Taenia solium* in a rural community in Mexico. *American Journal of Tropical Medicine and Hygiene*, 1997, 56(2):127-132.

248. Kachani M et al. Public health education/importance and experience from the field. Educational impact of community-based ultrasound screening surveys. *Acta Tropica*, 2003, 85(2):263-269.

249. Matibag GC et al. A pilot study on the usefulness of information and education campaign materials in enhancing the knowledge, attitude and practice on rabies in rural Sri Lanka. *Journal of Infection in Developing Countries*, 2009, 3(1):55-64.

250. Gonzalez AE et al. Control of *Taenia solium*. *Acta Tropica*, 2003, 87(1)103-109.

251. *The state of food and agriculture. Livestock in the balance*. Rome, Food and Agriculture Organization of the United Nations, 2009.

252. Pondja A et al. Prevalence and risk factors of porcine cysticercosis in Angonia District, Mozambique. *PLoS Neglected Tropical Diseases*, 2010, 4(2):594.

253. Chomel BB. Control and prevention of emerging parasitic zoonoses. *International Journal for Parasitology*, 2008, 38(11):1211-1217.

254. Macpherson CN. Human behaviour and the epidemiology of parasitic zoonoses. *International Journal for Parasitology*, 2005, 35(11-12):1319-1331.

255. Nesbitt A et al. High-risk food consumption and food safety practices in a Canadian community. *Journal of Food Protection*, 2009, 72(12):2575-2586.

256. Hu GH et al. The role of health education and health promotion in the control of schistosomiasis: experiences from a 12-year intervention study in the Poyang Lake area. *Acta Tropica*, 2005, 96(2-3):232-241.

257. Joshi DD et al. Controlling *Taenia solium* in Nepal using the PRECEDE-PROCEED model. *The Southeast Asian Journal of Tropical Medicine and Public Health*, 2001, 32(Suppl 2):94-97.

258. Ngowi H et al. Implementation and evaluation of a health-promotion strategy for control of *Taenia solium* infections in northern Tanzania. *International Journal of Health Promotion and Education*, 2009, 47(1):24-34.

259. Green LW, Kreuter MW. *Health program planning: an educational and ecological approach. 4th ed.* New York, McGraw-Hill Higher Education, 2005.

260. Earl S, Carden S, Smutylo T. *Outcome mapping. Building learning and reflection into development programs*. Ottawa, International Development Research Centre (IDRC), 2001.

261. Nielsen-Bohlman L, Panzer AM, Kindig DA, eds. *Health literacy: a prescription to end confusion*. Washington DC, National Academies Press, 2004.

262. Nutbeam D. The evolving concept of health literacy. *Social Science and Medicine*, 2008, 67(12):2072-2078.

263. von Wagner C et al. Health literacy and health actions: a review and a framework from health psychology. *Health Education and Behavior*, 2009, 36(5):860-877.

264. Aagaard-Hansen J, Mwanga JR, Bruun B. Social science perspectives on schistosomiasis control in Africa: past trends and future directions. *Parasitology*, 2009, 136(13):1747-1758.

265. Nutbeam D. Health literacy as a public health goal: a challenge for contemporary health education and communication strategies into the 21st century. *Health Promotion International*, 2000, 15(3):259-267.

266. Lamine D et al., Feasibility of Onchocerciasis Elimination with Ivermectin Treatment in Endemic Foci in Africa: First Evidence from Studies in Mali and Senegal, *PLoS Neglected Tropical Diseases*, 2009, 3(7): e497.

267. Umur S. Prevalence and economic importance of cystic echinococcosis in slaughtered ruminants in Burdur, Turkey. *Journal of Veterinary Medicine, Infectious Diseases and Veterinary Public health*, 2003, 50(5):247-252.

268. Zinsstag J et al. Transmission dynamics and economics of rabies control in dogs and humans in an African city. *Proceedings of the National Academy of Sciences of the United States of America*, 2009, 106(35):14996-15001.

269. Rupprecht CE et al. Can rabies be eradicated? *Developmental Biology*, 2008, 131:95-121.

270. Mallewa M et al. Rabies encephalitis in malaria-endemic area, Malawi, Africa. *Emerging Infectious Diseases*, 2007, 13(1):136-139.

271. Rupprecht CE, Hanlon CA, Hemachudha T. Rabies re-examined. *The Lancet Infectious Diseases*, 2002, 2(6):327-343.

272. Lembo T et al. Evaluation of a direct, rapid immunohistochemical test for rabies diagnosis. *Emerging Infectious Diseases*, 2006, 12(2):310-313.

273. Kang B et al. Evaluation of a rapid immunodiagnostic test kit for rabies virus. *Journal of Virological Methods*, 2007, 145(1):30-36.

274. Nishizono A et al. A simple and rapid immunochromatographic test kit for rabies diagnosis. *Microbiology and Immunology*, 2008, 52(4):243-249.

275. Markotter W et al. Evaluation of a rapid immunodiagnostic test kit for detection of African lyssaviruses from brain material. *Journal of Veterinary Research*, 2009, 76:257–262.

276. Muller T et al. Development of a mouse monoclonal antibody cocktail for post-exposure rabies prophylaxis in humans. *PLoS Neglected Tropical Diseases*, 2009, 3(11):542.

277. *Human and dog rabies prevention and control: Report of the WHO/Bill & Melinda Gates Foundation Consultation, Annecy, France 7-9 Octoboer 2009*. Geneva, World Health Organization, 2010.

278. Kunda J. E*pidemiology of zoonoses in the context of brucellosis in Tanzania*. Edinburgh, University of Edinburgh, 2006.

279. Cadmus SI et al. *Mycobacterium bovis* and *M. tuberculosis* in goats, Nigeria. Emerging Infectious Diseases, 2009, 15(12):2066-2067.

Appendix 1

Membership of Disease-specific Reference Group on Zoonoses and Marginalized Infectious Diseases of Poverty (DRG 6)

	Names	Country	Expertise	Gender
CHAIR	Professor David Molyneux	United Kingdom	Parasitology/ epidemiology	M
CO-CHAIR	Dr Zuhair Hallaj	Syria	Clinical medicine/ epidemiology (infectious diseases)	M
MEMBERS	Professor Gerard Keusch	USA	Communicable diseases	M
	Professor Pilar Ramos-Jimenez	Philippines	Health Social Siences	F
	Dr Helena Ngowi	United Republic of Tanzania	Veterinary/public health	F
	Dr Sarah Cleaveland	USA/United Kingdom	Wildlife biology	F
	Dr Don McManus	United Kingdom/ Australia	Parasitology/ microbiology/ genomics and genetics	M
	Dr Hélèn Carabin	USA/ Canada	Health/agriculture economics	F
	Dr Eduardo Gotuzzo	Peru	Infectious diseases	M
	Dr Kamal Kar	India	Water and sanitation	M
	Dr Ana Sanchez	Honduras/ Canada	Parasitology	F
	Dr Amadou Garba	Niger	Clinical medicine (infectious diseases)	M

Appendix 2

Disease-specific and thematic reference groups (DRGs/TRGs), the think tank for infectious diseases of poverty and host countries

Reference group		Host institution and country
DRG1	Malaria	WHO country office, Cameroon
DRG2	Tuberculosis, leprosy and Buruli ulcer	WHO country office, Philippines
DRG3	Chagas disease, human African trypanosomiasis and leishmaniasis	WHO country offices, Sudan and Brazil
DRG4	Helminth infections	African Programme for Onchocerciasis Control (APOC), Burkina Faso
DRG5	Dengue and other emerging viral diseases of public health importance	WHO country office, Cuba
DRG6	Zoonoses and marginalized infectious diseases of poverty	WHO Regional Office for the Eastern Mediterranean, Egypt
TRG1	Social sciences and gender	WHO country office, Ghana
TRG2	Innovation and technology platforms for health interventions in infectious diseases of poverty	WHO country office, Thailand
TRG3	Health systems and implementation research	WHO country office, Nigeria
TRG4	Environment, agriculture and infectious diseases of poverty	WHO country office, China

Appendix 3

Think tank members

Professor Pedro Alonso, Director and Research Professor, Barcelona Centre for International Health Research (CRESIB), Barcelona, Spain

Professor Rose Leke, Head, Department of Microbiology, Immunology, Hematology and Infectious Diseases, Faculty of Medicine and Biomedical Sciences, University of Yaoundé, Yaoundé, Cameroon

Dr Joel Breman, Senior Scientific Adviser, Fogarty International Center, Division of International Epidemiology & Population Studies, National Institutes of Health, Bethesda, MD, USA

Professor Graham Brown, Foundation Director, Nossal Institute for Global Health, University of Melbourne, Carlton, Victoria, Australia

Dr Chetan Chitnis, Principal Investigator, International Centre for Genetic Engineering and Biotechnology (ICGEB), New Delhi, India

Professor Alan Cowman, Researcher, Walter and Eliza Hall Institute of Medical Research, Parkville, Victoria, Australia

Professor Abdoulaye Djimdé, Research Scientist, Chief of Laboratory, Malaria Research and Training Center (MRTC), University of Bamako, and Malian EDCTP Senior Fellow, Bamako, Mali

Dr Sócrates Herrera Valencia, Director, Caucaseco Scientific Research Center (SRC), Instituto de Inmunología del Valle, Malaria Vaccine & Drug Development Centre, Universidad del Valle, Cali, Colombia

Professor Marcelo Jacobs-Lorena, Johns Hopkins School of Public Health, Department of Molecular Microbiology and Immunology, Malaria Research Institute, Baltimore, MD, USA

Dr Ramanan Laxminarayan, Director, Center for Disease Dynamics, Economics and Policy (CDDEP), Washington, DC, USA

Professor Rosanna Peeling, Chair of Diagnostics Research, London School of Hygiene & Tropical Medicine, Department of Infectious and Tropical Diseases, Clinical Research Unit, London, England

Professor Akintunde Sowunmi, University College Hospital, Malaria Research Laboratories, Institute of Advanced Medical Research and Training (IAMRAT), Ibadan, Nigeria

Dr Sarah Volkman, Senior Research Scientist, Harvard School of Public Health, Department of Immunology and Infectious Diseases, Boston, MA, USA

Dr Tim Wells, Chief Scientific Officer, Medicines for Malaria Venture (MMV), Geneva, Switzerland

Professor Gavin Churchyard, Chief Executive Officer, Aurum Institute, Johannesburg, South Africa

Professor Charles Yu, Medical Director and Vice President for Medical Services, De La Salle Health Sciences Institute, Vice-Chancellor's Office for Mission, Cavite, Philippines

Dr Madhukar Pai, Assistant Professor, McGill University, Department of Epidemiology, Biostatistics & Occupational Health, Montreal, Quebec, Canada

Dr Ann M. Ginsberg, Senior Advisor, Global Alliance for TB Drug Development, New York, NY, USA

Dr Jintana Ngamvithayapong-Yanai, President, TB/HIV Research Foundation, Chiang Rai, Thailand

Professor Laura C. Rodrigues, Head, Department of Epidemiology and Population Health, London School of Hygiene & Tropical Medicine, London, England

Professor Martien Borgdorff, Head, Cluster Infectious Diseases, Municipal Health Service of Amsterdam and Professor of Epidemiology, University of Amsterdam, Amsterdam, Netherlands

Professor Biao Xu, Director of Tuberculosis Research Center, Professor of Epidemiology and Deputy Chair, Department of Epidemiology, School of Public Health, Fudan University, Shanghai, China

Dr Francis Adatu Engwau, Programme Manager, National Tuberculosis/Leprosy Programme, Kampala, Uganda

Dr Anthony David Harries, Senior Advisor, Director, Department of Research, London School of Hygiene & Tropical Medicine. University of London, London, England

Dr Timothy Paul Stinear, Head of Research Group NHMRC, R. Douglas Wright Research Fellow, Department of Microbiology and Immunology, University of Melbourne, Parkville, Victoria, Australia

Dr Helen Ayles, Director, ZAMBART Project, London School of Hygiene & Tropical Medicine, ZAMBART, Ridgeway Campus, University of Zambia, Lusaka, Zambia

Professor Diana Lockwood, Department of Infectious and Tropical Diseases, London School of Hygiene & Tropical Medicine, London, England

Professor Ken Stuart, President Emeritus & Founder, Seattle Biomedical Research Institute, Seattle, WA, USA

Professor Maowia M. Mukhtar, Institute of Endemic Diseases, Department of Molecular Biology, University of Khartoum, Khartoum, Sudan

Professor Bianca Zingales, Instituto de Quimica, Universidade de São Paulo, São Paulo, Brazil

Professor Marleen Boelaert, Head, Department of Public Health, Institut de Médecine Tropical, Epidemiology & Disease Control Unit, Department of Public Health, Antwerp, Belgium

Ms Marianela Castillo-Riquelme, Departamento de Economía de la Salud, DIPLAS, Subsecretaría de Salud Publica, Ministerio de Salud de Chile, Santiago, Chile

Professor Mike J. Lehane, Professor of Molecular Entomology and Parasitology, Liverpool School of Tropical Medicine, Liverpool, England

Professor Pascal Lutumba, Institut National de Recherche Bio-Médicale, Kinshasa University, Democratic Republic of the Congo

Dr Enock Matovu, Senior Lecturer, Faculty of Veterinary Medicine, Makerere University, Department of Veterinary, Parasitology and Microbiology, Kampala, Uganda

Dr David Sacks, Head, Intracellular Parasite Biology Section, National Institutes of Health, National Institute of Allergy and Infectious Diseases, Laboratory of Parasitic Diseases, Bethesda, MD, USA

Dr Sergio Alejandro Sosa-Estani, Head, Service of Epidemiology, Instituto de Efectividad Clinica y Sanitaria, Buenos Aires, Argentina

Dr Shyam Sundar, Department of Medicine, Institute of Medical Sciences, Banaras Hindu University, Varanasi, India

Professor Rick L. Tarleton, Distinguished Research Professor, Center for Tropical & Emerging Global Diseases, Coverdell Center for Biomedical Research, University of Georgia, Athens, GA, USA

Professor Alon Warburg, Professor of Vector Biology and Parasitology, The Kuvin Center for the Study of Infectious and Tropical Diseases, Faculty of Medicine, Hebrew University, Einkerem, Israel

Dr Sara Lustigman, Head, Laboratory of Molecular Parasitology, Lindsley F. Kimball Research Institute, New York Blood Center, New York, NY, USA

Dr Boakye Boatin, Noguchi Memorial Institute for Medical Research, University of Ghana, Legon, Accra, Ghana

Dr Guojing Yang, Vice Head, Department of Schistosomiasis Control, Jiangsu Institute of Parasitic Diseases, Wuxi, China

Dr Rashida M.D.R. Barakat, High Institute of Public Health, Alexandria University, Alexandria, Egypt

Dr Maria Gloria Basanez, Professor of Neglected Tropical Diseases, Department of Infectious Disease Epidemiology, Faculty of Medicine, Imperial College, London, England

Dr KwablahAwadzi, Onchocerciasis Chemotherapy Research Centre, Hohoe Hospital, Hohoe, Ghana

Professor Banchob Sripa, Division of Experimental Pathology, Department of Pathology, Faculty of Medicine, KhonKaen University, KhonKaen, Thailand

Professor Warwick Grant, Head of Genetics, School of Molecular Sciences, Genetic Department, La Trobe University, Bundoora, Victoria, Australia

Professor Roger K. Prichard, Professor of Biotechnology, Institute of Parasitology, McGill University, Ste Anne de Bellevue, Quebec, Canada

Professor Hector Hugo Garcia, Department of Microbiology and Cysticercosis Unit, Instituto de Ciencias Neurologicas, Universidad Peruana Cayetano Heredia, Lima, Peru

Dr James McCarthy, Group Leader, Clinical Tropical Medicine, Queensland Institute of Medical Research, University of Queensland, Herston, Queensland, Australia

Professor Kouakou Eliezer N'Goran, Professeur de Biologie, Laboratoire de Zoologie et de Biologie Animale, Université de Cocody, Abidjan, Côte d'Ivoire

Dr Andréa Gazzinelli, School of Nursing, Federal University of Minas Gerais, Belo Horizonte, MG, Brazil

Dr Jeremy Farrar, Director, Oxford University Clinical Research Unit in Viet Nam, The Hospital for Tropical Diseases, Ho Chi Minh City, Viet Nam

Professor Maria Guzman, Head, Virology Department, Instituto de Medicina Tropical "Pedro Kouri", Havana, Cuba

Dr Natarajan Arunachalam, Senior Grade Deputy Director, Centre for Research in Medical Entomology, Indian Council of Medical Research, Madurai, India

Dr Duane Gubler, Professor, Director, Asia-Pacific Institute of Tropical Medicine and Infectious Diseases, John A Burns School of Medicine, University of Hawaii, Honolulu, HI, USA

Dr Sirirpen Kalayanarooj, Queen Sirikit National Institute of Child Health, Bangkok, Thailand

Dr Linda Lloyd, Director, Center for Research, The Institute for Palliative Medicine at San Diego Hospice, San Diego, CA, USA

Dr Lucy Chai See Lum, Associate Professor of Paediatrics, Department of Paediatrics, Faculty of Medicine, University of Malaya Medical Centre, Kuala Lumpur, Malaysia

Dr Amadou Sall, Chef de l'Unité des Arbovirus et Virus des Fièvres hémorragiques, Insitut Pasteur de Dakar, Arboviruses Unit/WHO Collaborating and Conference Centre, Dakar, Senegal

Dr Eric Martinez Torres, Instituto de Medicina Tropical Pedro Kouri, Havana, Cuba

Dr Philip J. McCall, Vector Group, Liverpool School of Tropical Medicine, Liverpool, England

Professor Derek Cummings, Assistant Professor, Department of Epidemiology, Bloomberg School of Public Health, Johns Hopkins University, Baltimore, MD, USA

Dr Hongjie Yu, Deputy Director, Professor, Office for Disease Control and Emergency Response, Chinese Center for Disease Control and Prevention, Beijing, China

Professor David Molyneux, Senior Professorial Fellow, Liverpool School of Tropical Medicine, Liverpool, England

Dr Zuhair Hallaj, Senior Consultant on Communicable Diseases, WHO Regional Office for the Eastern Mediterranean, Cairo, Egypt

Dr Gerald T. Keusch, Professor of International Health and of Medicine, Boston University, Boston, MA, USA

Dr Pilar Ramos-Jimenez, Philippine NGO Council on Population, Health and Welfare, Pasay City, Philippines

Professor Donald Peter McManus, National Health and Medical Research Council of Australia, Senior Principal Research Fellow, Head of Molecular Parasitology Laboratory, Queensland Institute of Medical Research, Brisbane, Queensland, Australia

Dr Eduardo Gotuzzo, Director, Instituto de Medicina Tropical "Alexander von Homboldt", Universidad Peruana Cayetano Heredia, Lima, Peru

Dr Kamal Kar, Chairman, CLTS Foundation, Calcutta, India

Dr Ana Sanchez, Associate Professor, Department of Community Health Sciences, Brock University, St. Catharines, Ontario, Canada

Dr Amadou Garba, Director, Réseau International Schistosomose, Environnement, Aménagement et Lutte (RISEAL), Niamey, Niger

Dr Helena Ngowi, Department of Veterinary Medicine and Public Health, Sokoine University of Agriculture, Mongoro, United Republic of Tanzania

Dr Sarah Cleaveland, Reader, Division of Ecology and Evolutionary Biology, University of Glasgow, Glasgow, Scotland

Dr Hélène Carabin, University of Oklahoma, Oklahoma Health Sciences Center, Oklahoma City, OK, USA

Professor Barbara McPake, Director and Professor, Institute for International Health and Development, Queen Margaret University, Edinburgh, Scotland

Dr Margaret Gyapong, Director, Dodowa Health Research Centre, Ghana Health Service, Dodowa, Ghana

Professor Juan Arroyo Laguna, Profesor Principal del Departamento Académico de Salud y Ciencias Sociales, FASPA-UPCH, Universidad Pruana Cayetano Heredia, Lima, Peru

Professor Sarah Atkinson, Reader, Department of Geography, University of Durham, Science Laboratories, Durham, England

Professor Rama Baru, Professor, Centre of Social Medicine and Community Health, Jawaharlal Nehru University, New Delhi, India

Professor Otto Nzapfurundi Chabikuli, Regional Technical Director, Africa Region with Family Health International (FHI360), Pretoria, South Africa

Professor Kalinga Tudor Silva, Senior Professor, Faculty of Arts, University of Peradeniya and Executive Director, International Centre for Ethnic Studies, Kandy, Sri Lanka

Professor Charles Hongoro, Research Director, Policy Analysis Unit, Human Sciences Research Council, Pretoria, South Africa

Professor Mario Mosquera-Vasquez, Associate Professor, Departamento de Comunicación Social, Universidad del Norte, Barranquilla, Colombia

Professor Chuma Jane Mumbi, Research Fellow, Kenya Medical Research Institute, Wellcome Trust Research Programme, Kilifi, Kenya Professor Helle Samuelsen, Head, Department of Anthropology, University of Copenhagen, Copenhagen, Denmark

Professor Sally Theobald, Liverpool School of Tropical Medicine, Liverpool, England

Professor Mitchell Weiss, Professor and Head of the Department of Public Health and Epidemiology Swiss Tropical Institute, Basel, Switzerland

Professor Yongyuth Yuthavong, Senior Researcher, National Centre for Genetic Engineering and Biotechnology (BIOTEC), Bangkok, Thailand

Professor Simon Croft, Professor of Parasitology, Department of Infectious and Tropical Diseases, London School of Hygiene and Tropical Medicine, London, England

Professor Rama Baru, Professor, Centre of Social Medicine and Community Health, Jawaharlal Nehru University, New Delhi, India

Professor Sanaa Botros, Manager of Training and Consultation Unit, Theodor Bilharz Research Institute, Imbaba, Giza, Egypt

Dr Mary Jane Cardosa, Director, Institute of Health and Community Medicine, University Malaysia Sarawak, Kota, Malaysia

Professor Simon Efange, Professor of Chemistry, University of Buea, Buea, Cameroon

Dr Vish Nene, Director of Biotechnology Thematic Group, International Livestock Research Institute, Nairobi, Kenya

Dr Antonio Oliveira-Dos-Santos, Medical Affairs Director, Genzyme, Rio de Janeiro, Brazil

Professor Paul Reider, Department of Chemistry, Princeton University, Princeton, NJ, USA

Dr Giorgio Roscigno, Former Chief Executive Officer, Foundation for Innovative New Diagnostics, Budé, Geneva, Switzerland

Professor Anthony So, Director, Terry Stanford Institute of Public Health Policy, Duke University, Durham, NC, USA

Professor Ming-Wei Wang, Director, The National Centre for Drug Screening, Shanghai, China

Dr Miguel Angel González-Block, Executive Director, Centre for Health Systems Research, National Institute of Public Health, Cuernavaca, Mexico

Professor Olayiwola Akinsonwon Erinosho, Executive Secretary at Health Reform Foundation of Nigeria (HERFON), Abuja, Nigeria

Dr Charles Collins, Honorary Senior Research Fellow, University of Birmingham, Birmingham, England

Dr Dyna Arhin, Associate Consultant, Public Health Action Support Team (PHAST), Faculty of Medicine, Imperial College London, England

Dr Abbas Bhuiya, Senior Social Scientist, Head, Poverty and Health Programme and Social and Behavioural Sciences Unit, Public Health Sciences Division, ICDDR,B, Mohakhali, Dhaka, Bangladesh

Dr Celia Maria de Almeida, Senior Researcher and Professor in Health Policy and Health Systems Organization, Health Administration and Planning Department, Escola Nacional de Saude Publica-ENSP/Fiocruz, Rio de Janeiro, Brazil

Professor Barun Kanjilal, Professor, Indian Institute of Health Management Research, Jaipur, India

Dr Joseph Kasonde, Executive Director, Zambia Forum for Health Research, Lusaka, Zambia

Dr Dorothée Kinde-Gazard, Minister of Health, The National AIDS Control Probramme (PNLS), Cotonou, Benin

Dr Samuel Wanji, Research Foundation for Tropical Diseases and the Environment, Buea, Cameroon

Professor Anthony McMichael, Professor, National Centre for Epidemiology and Population Health, Australian National University, Canberra, ACT, Australia

Professor Xiao-Nong Zhou, Director, National Institute of Parasitic Disease, China Centers for Disease Control, Shanghai, China

Professor Corey Bradshaw, Director of Ecological Modelling, The Environment Institute and School of Earth & Environmental Sciences, University of Adelaide, Adelaide, Western Australia, Australia

Dr Stuart Gillespie, Director, RENEWAL, Coordinator, Agriculture and Health Research Platform, International Food Policy Research Institute (IFPRI), c/o UNAIDS, Geneva, Switzerland

Dr Suad M. Sulaiman, Health & Environment Adviser, Khartoum, Sudan

Professor James A. Trostle, Professor of Anthropology, Anthropology Department, Trinity College, Hartford, CT, USA

Dr Jürg Ützinger, Assistant Professor, Department of Public Health and Epidemiology, Swiss Tropical Institute, Basel, Switzerland

Professor Bruce Wilcox, Professor and Director of the Global Health Program at the University of Hawaii, Honolulu, HI, USA

Dr Guojing Yang, Assistant Professor (Principal Investigator), Dept. Schistosomiasis Control, Jiangsu Institute of Parasitic Diseases, Jiangsu Province, China

Appendix 4

Distribution of the Think Tank leadership (co-Chairs)

Think tank co-chairs and host countries

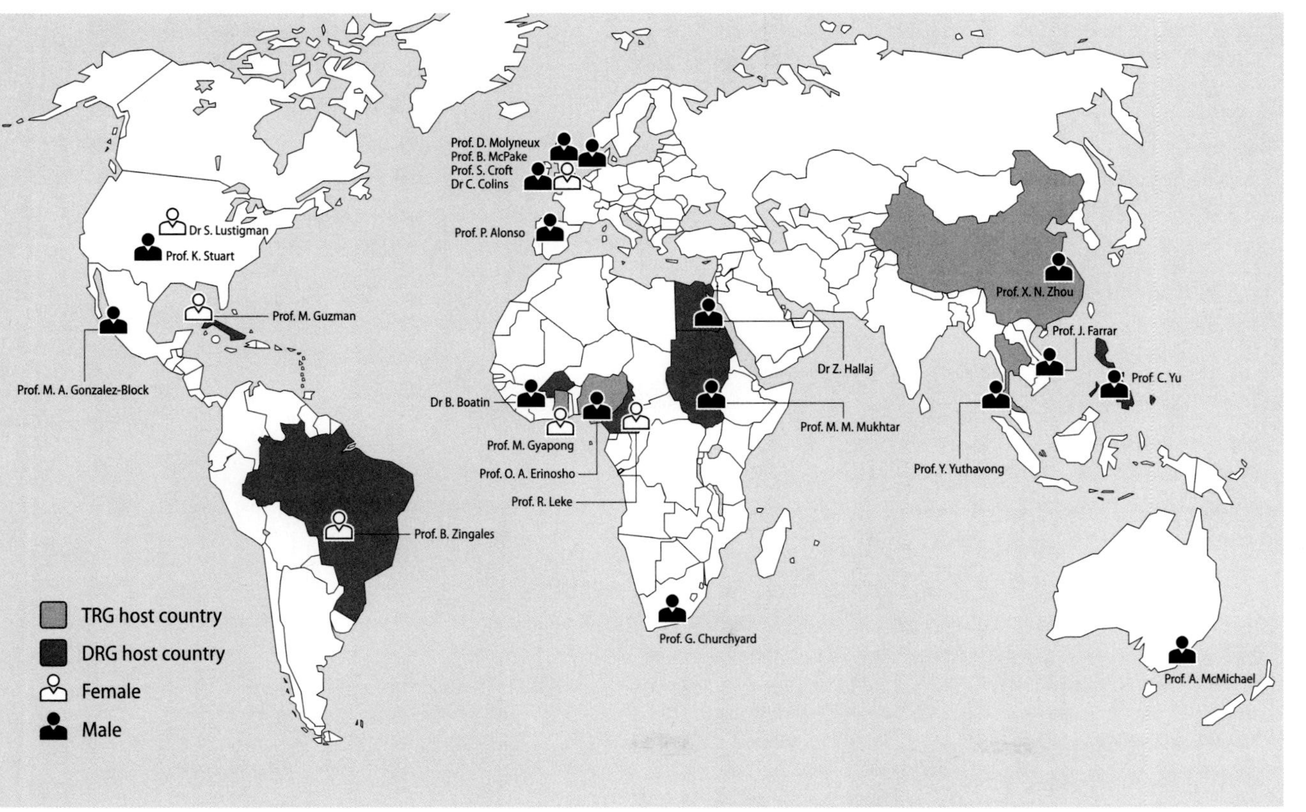

TRG: Thematic Reference Group
DRG: Disease-specific Reference Group